Sexually Transmitted Diseases

(Venereal Diseases)

Sexually Transmitted Diseases
(Venereal Diseases)

5th Edition

Virendra N Sehgal
MD FNASc FAMS FRAS (London)

Visiting Professor
Skin Institute and School of Dermatology

Consultant
Dermato-venereologist

Former
Director-Professor and Head
Department of Dermatology and Venereology
Maulana Azad Medical College and Associated
Lok Nayak Jay Prakash Hospital, New Delhi

Principal/Medical Superintendent/
Director-Professor Dermatology and Venereology
Lady Hardinge Medical College, New Delhi

Director-Professor Dermatology/
Venereology/Medical Superintendent
University College of Medical Sciences and
Associated Guru Teg Bahadur Hospital
Delhi

JAYPEE

JAYPEE BROTHERS MEDICAL PUBLISHERS
The Health Sciences Publisher
New Delhi | London

Jaypee Brothers Medical Publishers (P) Ltd

Headquarters
EMCA House
23/23-B, Ansari Road, Daryaganj
New Delhi 110 002, India
Landline: +91-11-23272143, +91-11-23272703
+91-11-23282021, +91-11-23245672
E-mail: jaypee@jaypeebrothers.com

Corporate Office
4838/24, Ansari Road, Daryaganj
New Delhi 110 002, India
Phone: +91-11-43574357
Fax: +91-11-43574314
E-mail: jaypee@jaypeebrothers.com

Overseas Office
J.P. Medical Ltd.
83, Victoria Street, London
SW1H 0HW (UK)
Phone: +44-20 3170 8910
E-mail: info@jpmedpub.com

EU GPSR Authorised Representative
Logos Europe, 9 rue Nicolas Poussin
17000, La Rochelle, France
Phone: +33 (0) 6 67 93 73 78
E-mail: contact@logoseurope.eu

Website: www.jaypeebrothers.com
Website: www.jaypeedigital.com

Inquiries for bulk sales may be solicited at: jaypee@jaypeebrothers.com

Sexually Transmitted Diseases (Venereal Diseases)

First Edition: 1978
Second Edition: 1987
Third Edition: 1993
Fourth Edition: 2003
Reprint: *2006*
Fifth Edition: 2010
Reprint: **2026**

ISBN 978-81-8448-954-5

Printed in India

Preface to the Fifth Edition

Once again, Almighty bestowed an opportunity to bring about the current innovation in the text. Treatment perceptions of STDs were considered paramount, for which 'World Health Organization (WHO) guidelines for the treatment of STDs' were taken stock of. Accordingly, they were imbibed in the respective disease(s) to facilitate their use in day-to-day practice. Furthermore, it was considered worthwhile to provide an acceptable alternative. 'Center for Disease Control and Prevention (CDC) guidelines for the treatment of sexually transmitted infections (appendix 10)* is a viable document for the purpose. Besides, references are updated in accordance to 'Pubmed, US National Library of Medicine National Institutes of Health,' and are arranged to match the modified Vancour style. Surely, the current edition should evoke renewed interest in the subject amongst under- and postgraduates, and practicing physicians.

The instant assistance given by Dr Sambit N Bhattacharya, Professor and Head, Department of Dermatology, STD and Leprosy, UCMS and GTB Hospital, Delhi and Dr Vibhu Mendiratta, Professor and Head, Department of Dermatology, STD and Leprosy, Lady Harding Medical College, and Associated Smt Sucheta Kriplani and Kalawati Saran Children Hospitals, New Delhi, is greatly appreciated. My computer assistant Shailender Sehgal laboriously executed the organization of the final version of the text of the book.

Virendra N Sehgal

*Anonymous. Sexually transmitted diseases treatment guidelines, 2002. Centers for Disease Control and Prevention. MMWR Recomm Rep 2002; 51:1-78.

Preface to the First Edition

The book is based on the didactic lectures and clinical demonstrations on venereal diseases, which the author has been giving to undergraduate and also to postgraduate students. The contents of the text conform to the curricula for undergraduates of different universities. It is concise, succinct, and aptly illustrated. Emphasis has, however, been placed on the classic clinical features of common venereal diseases. Essentials of diagnostic procedures, the treatment, and also follow-up have been clearly outlined. The present challenges of these diseases are described under epidemiology, while their control status, and prospective planning for prevention is delineated separately. The book is written primarily for the students; it is hoped, however, that it may be useful also to the practising physicians, for venereal diseases are sparingly described in books of medicine.

Virendra N Sehgal

Contents

Chapter 1

History Taking

INTRODUCTION

History taking and the physical examination of a venereal disease patient is similar to that in general medicine. This examination should be preceded by reassurance and evincing confidence in him. This is imperative, for venereal diseases are invariably associated with some psychological aberrations. An endeavor should always be, to form an absolute picturesque genesis of the relevant disease. In order to accomplish this objective, an emphasis should be laid on the following points while forming the history.

Marital status; single/married/divorcee/ or a widow/widower. Occupation, whether living at home or away from home and patient's temporary and permanent address. Recent history of sexual exposure should be taken in great detail. The exact dates of exposure and its particulars such as, place of exposure; whether it was heterosexual or homosexual; contraceptives used, if any; details of intercourse; genital/orogenital/oral: history of trauma to genitalia and amount of money paid, should be recorded. It is necessary to ask about the health of sexual partner incorporating whether she was having vaginal discharge and/or genital sores at the exposure time, and details of each should be noted.

Venereal disease patient usually presents with a complaint of either discharge per urethra and/or genital sore. In patients presenting with discharge per urethra and burning micturition, the following details should be noted: amount—copious/scanty; color—milky white/yellowish/bloodstained; consistency—thin watery/thick, and its relation to micturition. History of morning gleet, dull pain in the abdomen/perineum, sense of fullness of rectum and pain during defecation should also be elicited.

In patients presenting with genital sore(s), further details namely number of lesions; whether they are painful or painless; any preceding erythema and/or burning sensation; discharge from the sore and swelling confined to glans, prepuce or both, should be recorded. In patients presenting with genital growth, it is necessary to ask whether it bleeds on touch, and its rate of progress. Further, history of constitutional features and/or skin lesions may be contributory. The incubation period in particular may be recorded, as it may be very useful for arriving at a diagnosis. The incubation period in tropics, is as follows: gonorrhea and chancroid (2-5 days); syphilis (9-90 days); herpes genitalis (4-5 days); venereal warts (6-32 weeks); lymphogranuloma venereum (3 days-3 weeks); donovanosis (8-80 days) and non-specific urethritis (8-14 days).

Past history of venereal disease(s) and response to treatment should also be enquired. Personal history includes details about education, occupation, monthly income and addiction (alcohol/narcotics). In married patients, the date of last marital exposure, relation with the spouse and frequency of sexual intercourse, should be enquired. When relevant, enquire about health of the parents, siblings and causes of death, if any, in the family.

In female cases menstrual history is recorded. The obstetric history is noted in detail. The number of living children and their health, the causes of death, if any, and dates of any miscarriages, abortions or stillbirths, is important.

CLINICAL EXAMINATION

The patients should always be examined in daylight if possible. The genitalia are examined for any discharge, inflammation, edema, erosions, ulcers, warts or rashes. In case the prepuce is phimotic, the subpreputial discharge should be cleaned with a moist saline gauze and the prepuce is retracted as far back as possible. Examination of the genitalia should include the glans, coronal sulcus, external urethral meatus, shaft, scrotum, and pubic region. Other sites namely the inguinal, perianal regions, thighs, buttocks and breasts are also inspected. All mucous membranes are examined in detail.

The details of urethral discharge are recorded as amount; color; consistency; whether blood-stained or not; any associated redness and swelling of external urethral meatus. The following details of ulcers are then noted; number—single/multiple; size; shape—irregular/circular; borders—clear cut/everted/undermined/inflammatory; depth—superficial/deep; floor—clean/covered with necrotic material/having healthy granulation tissue; tenderness; induration and tendency to bleed on touch. The inguinal, external iliac, epitrochlear, axillary and cervical group of lymph nodes are also examined and their details noted as unilateral/bilateral; single/multiple; discrete/matted; consistency; tenderness; mobility; erythema of overlying skin and fixity to surrounding tissues.

The female patients should be examined in lithotomy position, in the presence of a female attendant, after taking consent of the patient. The abdomen is palpated for signs of tenderness and presence of scars. The pubic hair are examined for the presence of lice. The perineum, vulva, labia majora, labia minora and fourchette are examined for any discharge, signs of inflammation, edema,erosion, ulcers, warts or rashes. The labia are separated, the urethra examined and the Bartholin's glands palpated. After that a Cuscos bivalve speculum is passed inside the vagina and vaginal portion of the cervix is inspected. This examination should not be performed in a virgin. In children and virgins, the cervix is visualised with the ophthalmoscope for impacted foreign body or any other abnormality. The cervix is examined for any discharge and its character noted. After cleaning the discharge, the cervix is examined for any erosion/ulceration. As the speculum is being gradually withdrawn, the vaginal walls are inspected for any inflammation, cheesy plaques of candidosis and vaginal discharge. The details of discharge and ulcers are noted as in male patients. The smell of vaginal discharge, in particular, should be noted for this discharge in consequence to *Trichomonas vaginalis* is foul smelling and may be the presenting complaint. In addition pH of the discharge is worth recording. The fornices, the uterus and its appendages are then palpated. The movement of the cervix elicits marked tenderness in presence of pelvic inflammatory disease (PID). This sign is called *Chandelier's sign*. The urethra is massaged with the finger forward along the anterior vaginal wall. Any discharge from the urethra or paraurethral glands of Skene is noted. Examination for the extra-genital lesions, mucosa and lymph nodes is done as in males. A rectal smear and a throat swab should be taken whenever indicated.

The systemic examination must include details of the skin and mucosal surface, lymph nodes, joints, central nervous system, cardiovascular and respiratory system. An ophthalmic examination should also be done.

OFFICE PROCEDURES

Two Glass Test

The two glass test is done to assess the status of urethra. It gives a fair index of spread of gonococcal infection. The patient is asked to pass urine in two separate glasses, half in each glass. In case of urine being hazy in the first glass, it suggests anterior urethritis, while in the second, it indicates that infection has spread to the posterior urethra.

Prostatic Bassage

It is a vital component of clinical examination and is usually performed 28 days after adequate and specific treatment for urethritis. It should be undertaken in cases where past history of discharge per urethra; burning, frequency or difficulty in micturition, heaviness in lower abdomen and sense of fullness of rectum is experienced. It is also indicated in cases of posterior urethritis, where the second glass (in two glass test), is hazy. Further, it is imperative to prepare a urethral smear and then the patient is asked to void the urine before the prostatic massage is undertaken.

The object of the prostatic massage is to express the prostatic fluid from the gland into the posterior urethra, from where it will pass into anterior urethra and can be collected at the urinary meatus. After evacuating the bowels, the patient is placed in the knee-elbow position. The perianal region is inspected for piles, ulcers or growth. The patient should be told about what is to be done. He is also instructed to open his mouth and breathe smoothy. A gloved index finger lubricated with vaseline is kept at the anal opening and gentle pressure is exerted until the finger gradually slips into the rectum. The finger is then passed over the prostate till the superior border is felt. Its size, shape, consistency, state of overlying mucosa, surface (whether regular or not) and presence of tenderness, is noted. The groove between prostate and the seminal vesicles, is also felt. The condition of median groove is noted. Massage is undertaken only if there is no evidence of acute infection. The finger is gently passed above the lateral edge of the right lobe and firmly brought down in a direction parallel to the midline. Two other strokes are made with the finger medially. The same procedure is used on the left lobe. As a result the prostatic secretion is expressed into the urethra. Finally, the finger is brought down in the midline twice, so as to express the fluid through the sphincter into the penile urethra. During this period the patient feels a desire to urine and the secretions from urethral meatus are collected on clean glass slides for laboratory examination. Alternatively prostatic massage may be performed by stroking it from either side in a transverse direction.

Gram's Stain

The smear from the material is prepared with the platinum loop, it is dried and fixed by passing over the flame. It is stained with 0.5 percent methyl violet (crystal violet) solution for 20-30 seconds. The excess stain is poured off and Lugol's iodine solution is added to wash away methyl violet. Iodine is allowed to act for 30-60 seconds. Lugol's iodine is washed repeatedly with absolute alcohol until the color ceases to come out of the preparation. Later the smear is washed with water and counter stained with 0.5 percent safranine or neutral red for 30-60 seconds. Again it is washed with water and dried in between blotting papers. The stained smear is now ready for microscopic examination.

Wet Preparation

Wet preparations are useful to demonstrate *Candida albicans* and *Trichomonas vaginalis*. The method adopted for the collection of material, however, differs.

Candida albicans

For its demonstration the scraping or discharge is collected on a clean glass slide, to which a drop of KOH (10-20 percent) is added. After a short interval, the slide is examined under the light microscope for the spores or pseudomycelia.

Trichomonas vaginalis

Here again the discharge is collected on a glass slide. It may either be instantly examined or a drop of normal saline is added, before undertaking the examination. The morphology or motility can well be seen under light or dark-ground microscope.

Dark Ground Examination

The material for the dark ground examination for *Treponema pallidum* is collected, by applying an edge of the cover slip to the lesions such as primary chancre, condylomata lata, mucous membrane patches, after bathing them with normal saline. While the material from the lymph glands is collected by injecting a little quantity of normal saline into the glands, and aspirating it. This material too is taken on a cover slip which is later placed on a thin slide and examined under the dark-ground microscope.

Serological Tests for Syphilis

At least one non-specific-VDRL, TPHA and one specific TPI/ FTA-ABS test should preferably be performed in each case.

Tissues Smear for Donovan Bodies

After thorough clearning of the lesion, a small piece of granulomatous tissues is removed from the edge of a lesion with a forceps. The blood from the tissue is absorbed in a filter paper and an imprint of the tissue is made on a glass slide. The smear is dried, fixed, and stained with Giemsa's stain. The characteristic Donovan bodies are located in the mononuclear cells and are usually recognised by their "Safety pin" appearance, produced by the bipolar distribution of the chromatin material. In early cases the Donovan bodies may show no capsule. Occasionally, Donovan bodies may be seen lying extracellularly, consequent to rupture of a heavily parasitised mononuclear cell.

Chapter 2

Epidemiology of Sexually Transmitted Diseases/Infections

INTRODUCTION

Sexually transmitted diseases have recently been replaced by a euphemistic term—Sexually transmitted diseases (STD). This has now been widely adopted all over the world. Several diseases form a part component of STD, but gonorrhea, chancroid, and syphilis are important, because of their higher prevalence and/or morbidity. Other venereal diseases such as *lymphogranuloma venereum* and *granuloma inguinale* are less frequently encountered, largely affecting groups at risk, living in poor socio-economic conditions. There are some infections like herpes progenitalis, tricho-moniasis, *condylomata acuminata, candidiasis, scabies,* and *pediculosis* which may also be transmitted sexually. Non-venereal treponematoses such as *yaws, endemic syphilis, bejel* and *pinta* are conventionally considered with *syphilis,* because they are clinically and immunologically interrelated.

The sexually transmitted diseases (STD) are of cosmopolitan distribution, infecting both sexes, occurring in developed as well as under-developed countries. *Gonorrhea* and *syphilis* are common all over the world, but other venereal diseases such as *chancroid, lymphogranuloma venereum* and *granuloma inguinale* are quite common in developing countries, while they are sporadic in developed countries. Similarly non-venereal treponematoses were/are endemic in some underdeveloped tropical and subtropical areas of the world, where poor living standards and hygiene compounded by climatic factors and humidity may determine their endemicity.

The incidence of venereal diseases is determined by various factors, built around an environmental, behavioral and ill-understood psychological background. These factors are exactly similar in all the countries of the world, rich or poor.

YOUTH COMPONENT (TEENAGERS) AND SEX

The sexually transmitted diseases are commonly seen in the sexually active age of 20-40 years. But now the average age of STD patients is getting younger every year, more patients are applying for treatment in the age group of 15-19 and 20-24 years. Higher incidence in this age group has been attributed to several factors such as early physical maturity due to better nutritional standards, exposure to sex stimulating literature displayed in magazines, radio and television media. The incidence of STD in young people is, therefore, mounting higher and higher in the world population as a whole.

Both men and women suffer from the disease, but apparently the incidence is higher in men, for they invariably apply for treatment. The actual incidence in women may be much higher than that is generally noticed in day-to-day practice. It is attributed to the silent (symptomless) nature of the disease amongst them, coupled with their unwillingness to report for treatment. Hence they constitute the established reservoir and a salient link in transmitting and perpetuating these diseases.

EMERGENCE OF PERMISSIVE SOCIETY

There has been a considerable change in the moral standards and attitude of the society towards sex—a global feature—leading to greater permissiveness. It has, therefore, removed the traditional inhibitions imposed by the religion and the society on the sexual behavior. Similarly, explicit erosion of family influence and parental authority on the youth, have further deteriorated the situation. All these factors have been responsible for the so-called sexual" "revolution", which has sparked off the worldwide increase in sexually transmitted diseases.

Role of Prostitution

Prostitutes

The traditional reservoir of venereal diseases (VD) infection—continue to play a dominant role in the spread of VD. The fast changing-heterogenous-pattern of prostitution namely the semi-prostitutes engaged in normal jobs to call girls, car-prowling girls, cabaret-girls and casual contacts like married women practising prostitution on the side, have added fresh dimensions to the existing problem. Moreover, the girl-friends are now fast replacing the traditional prostitutes as the source of contamination. On the other hand, prostitutes have divorced the "red light areas" to have wider ramifications in the rural as well as urban areas to evade the authority control and to get better returns of their profession. Consequently, the effective control and contact tracing of the reservoir have become extremely difficult.

Homosexual Practice

Another important factor in the spread of venereal diseases is the practice of homosexuality by a sizable number of people in the larger cities of the world—the passive agent, acting as a reservoir of infection.

Demographic Factors

The rapid and progressive increase in population, especially of younger age groups has led to a considerable increase in the number of venereal diseases patients. It is a phenomenon, which is apparent in the developing countries, all over the world. In developing countries, in particular, economic development has not been able to keep pace with the rapid growth of population, thus causing all round-strain-on the exchequer, including medical services. Consequently, it has caused mushroom growth of over crowded slums, formed of poor or inadequate sanitation, scarce water supply and poor housing. Hence, an ideal environment is formed for the maintenance of the reservoir and the spread of sexually transmitted diseases.

Family Planning

Various measures adopted to control the birth rate, e.g. the condoms, IUCDs and contraceptive pills have removed the fear of impregnation (pregnancy), and caused greater sex freedom for both men and women. Consequently, promiscuity is becoming a common phenomenon in the society. Hence, family planning is contributing in its own way to the increase of venereal diseases.

Population Movement

Persons engaged in occupations involving frequent travel are the high-risk groups. This includes sailors, truck drivers, sales representatives, tourists and pilgrims. It also holds good for army troops during war time.

Urbanization

The migration of youth from the rural to the industrial urban areas in search of vocations along with overcrowding, loneliness and anonymity, augments the chances of contracting venereal diseases. Furthermore, a higher incidence of venereal diseases is noted in affluent industrial workers. Additionally; venereal diseases are found predominantly in large cities, to which majority of young immigrants move and where casual encounters, prostitution, and homosexual practices are common. The spread of STD is also influenced by deteriorating areas of slums, amongst socially disorganized groups of low socioeconomic status. Moreover, the disproportion of male–female ratio in big cities may predispose to pre-and extramarital contacts.

Easy and Inadequate Treatment

Yet another and paradoxical reason for an increase in STD is the extreme simplicity and easy availability of treatment. The one-shot penicillin therapy of gonorrhea and syphilis has reduced the fear of the disease, and consequently increased the sexual contacts, under inadequate antibiotic cover, "antibiotics honeymoons" amongst the young. It is complemented by an emergence of antibiotic-resistant organisms—a feature frequently observed nowadays in response to inadequate and indiscriminate treatment.

Lack of Control Measures

In many developing countries and also in others, the governmental (official) facilities for the diagnosis, treatment, contact tracing, follow-up and health education are very meagre. The consequence is the

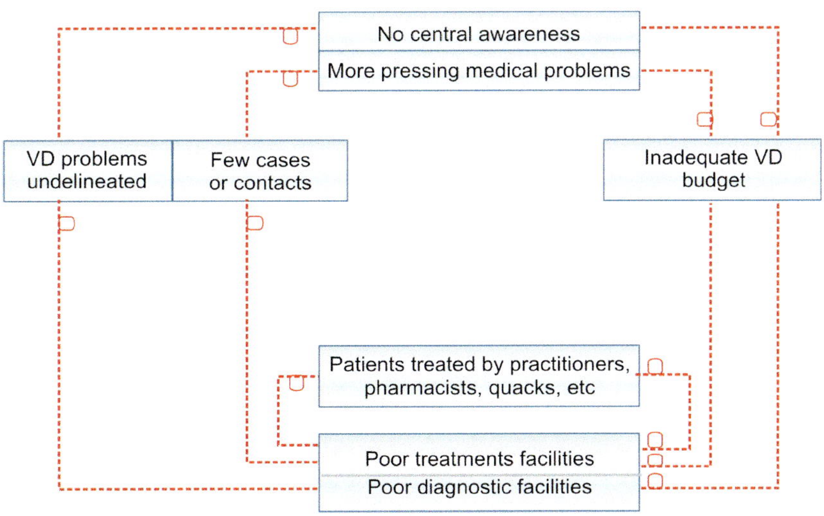

Fig. 2.1: 'Vicious circle', illustrating the sequence of events leading to the maintenance of reservoir and the perpetuation of STD in developing countries (Courtesy: RR Willcox, Brit J Vener Dis 1976;52:88)

setting in of the so-called 'vicious circle' (Fig 2.1), which illustrates the sequence of events leading to the maintenance of reservoir and the perpetuation of sexually transmitted diseases.

FURTHER READING

1. Anonymous. Venereal diseases and young people. A report by a Committee of the British Medical Association on the problem of venereal diseases. British Medical Association 1974.
2. Morton RS. 'Size and nature of the problems.' In: Morton RS, Harris JRW (Eds). Recent Advances in Sexually Transmitted Diseases', Edinburgh: Churchill Livingstone 1975.
3. Schofield M. Sexual Behavior of young people. London: Longman 1968.

Chapter 3

Applied Anatomy of the Genital Organs

INTRODUCTION

In order to understand the sexually transmitted diseases, it is worthwhile to review the applied anatomy of female and male genital organs.

FEMALE GENITAL ORGANS

External genital organs and their sagittal section is shown in Figures 3.1 and 3.2.

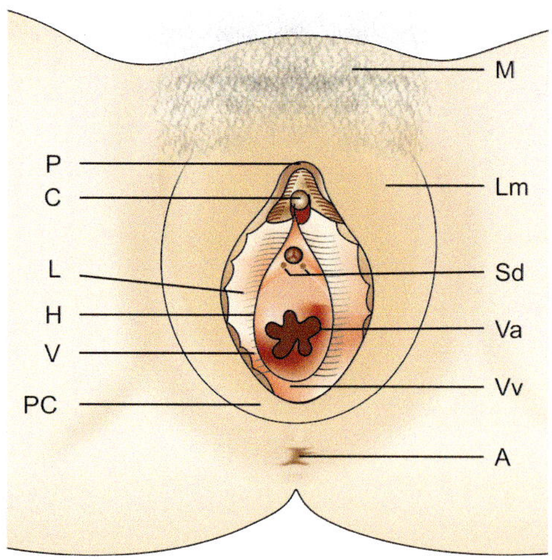

Fig. 3.1: External female genital organs, **P** prepuce; **C** clitoris; **L** labia minora; **H** hymen; **V** vestibule; **PC** posterior commissures; **M** mons veneris; **Lm** labia majora; **Sd** Skene's duct; **Va** vagina; A anus

Mons Veneris

The mons veneris is a median elevation in front of the symphysis pubis. It is covered with hair.

Labia Majora

Labia majora extend from the mons veneris to the fourchette. They consist of two longitudinal folds. Each fold has an outer and an inner surface. The outer surface is covered with hair and continues with the surrounding skin. The inner surface is smooth, hairless, pink in color and has many sebaceous glands.

Labia Minora

They are located on the inner surface of the labia majora and consist of two folds, one on either side. The skin is soft and has got abundant sebaceous glands. Anteriorly it divides into two folds. The anterior one passes in front of the clitoris and joins at the fourchette. The space between the two folds is the vestibule. It contains from above downwards the urinary meatus, the ducts of Bartholin's glands, and the vaginal opening.

Clitoris

It is a homologue of the male penis. It is an erectile structure situated in the midline between the anterior and posterior folds of the labia minora. It is covered by the prepuce. It is richly supplied by blood vessels and sensory nerves.

Bartholin's Glands

They correspond to Cowper's glands of the males. They are located under the superficial perineal fascia at the junction of upper two-third and lower one-third of labia minora. They are lined by columnar epithelium and are prone to get affected in gonorrheal infections. These glands open into the vestibule and secrete a clear mucus during sexual intercourse, which acts as a lubricant in the vulva.

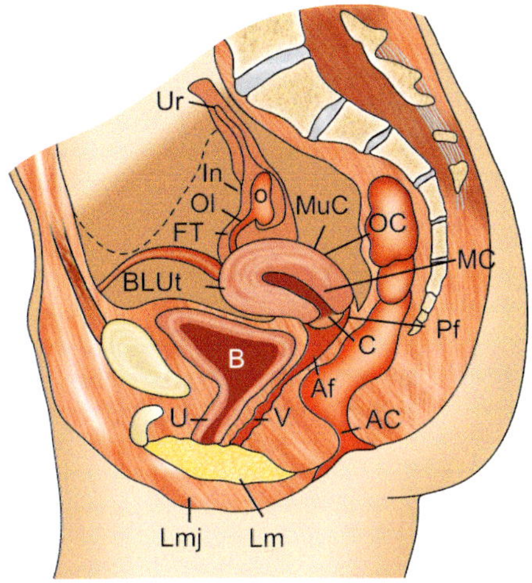

Fig. 3.2: Female genital organs, sagittal section. **MV** mons veneris; **Lmj** labia majora; **Lm** labia minora; **AC** anal canal; **U** urethra; **V** vagina; **C** cervix; **Af** anterior fornix; **pf** posterior fornix; **Ut** uterus; **MuC** muscular coat; **MC** mucous coat; **Oc** outer coat; **FT** fallopian tube; **Ol** ovarian ligament; **O** ovaries; **Ur** ureter; **B** bladder

Hymen

It is a longitudinal fold of mucous membrane of 0.25 cm thickness, partially blocking the vaginal orifice. It is composed of two layers of stratified squamous epithelium, with vascular connective tissue in between them.

Vagina

It is a canal located between the bladder and the urethra in front, and the rectum behind. It is obliquely placed. Its anterior wall is 9 cm and posterior wall is 14 cm long. The cervix projects into the roof of vagina. The concavity formed by the inver-sion of the uterus is divided by the protrud-ing cervix into anterior, posterior and two lateral fornices. The canal is lined by thick stratified squamous epithelium during the active reproductive period, while it is thin before puberty and atrophic after meno-pause. The vaginal pH is variable and is determined by *Doderlein's bacillus* and estrogenic hormones. The vagina is resistant to gonorrheal infection before puberty and at menopause, because of its alkaline pH during this period, but it is prone to get *Trichomonas vaginalis* infection. In adults the pH of the vagina is acidic, thereby reducing the chances for infection other than gonorrhea.

Uterus

It is suspended in the pelvis by the broad ligaments. It lies between the bladder and the rectum. The size of the uterus varies at different periods of life. It is 8 cm long, 5 cm broad and 2.2 cm thick in the nulliparous. The uterus is divided into the fundus, the body and the cervix. The junction of the body and the cervix is called isthmus. The fundus is the part lying above the line joining the uterine opening of the fallopian tubes, into the uterus. Microscopically, the body of the uterus is made up of mucous, muscular and serous coats. The mucous coat forms the endometrium. It is 2 mm thick. The muscular coat is composed of plain muscles as well as fibrous tissue in varying proportions at different periods of life. The serous coat forms the outer most covering, which continues with the peritoneal lining of the pelvic cavity.

Fallopian Tubes

Each tube is about 12 cm long. They are attached to the uterus at one end, while the other free end lies in the pelvic peritoneal cavity. Anatomically each tube is divided into the interstitial part, the isthmus and the ampullary parts. The small interstitial part is embedded in the uterine wall. It communicates with the uterine cavity by an opening 1-2 mm in diameter. The ostium is surrounded by tiny processes called finrbriae. Microscopically, it consists of an outer peritoneal coat, middle muscular and inner mucous membrane. The mucous membrane is lined by ciliated columnar epithelium. The tubes are the frequent seat of acute and chronic inflammatory diseases, which may either be secondary to ascending infection from the cervix or the uterus or by direct continuity or by the lymphatics.

Ovaries

These are two oval-shaped structures each measuring about 5 cm. They are attached to the posterior aspect of the broad ligament by a fold, the mesovarium, and also to the uterus by the ovarian ligament. They lie at the ostium of the fallopian tube.

Urethra

It is 4 cm long. It starts form the base of the bladder and extends downwards towards the external urinary meatus. It is located beneath the clitoris at the upper part of the vestibule. It is lined proximally by transitional epithelium and distally by stratified epithelium. Its mucous membrane contains small glands, which are lined by columnar epithelium. These glands open into the urethra.

Skene's Glands

These glands are situated on either side of external urinary meatus. They are lined by columnar epithelium. They may be affected in the genital infection.

Lymphatic Drainage

The lymphatics of the clitoris, the urethra and the vulva drain principally into the inguinal glands, which, in turn, are drained into the iliac and the hypogastric glands. The lymph vessels of the posterior third of the vulva and the fourchette anastomose freely with the lymphatics of the anus. The lymph vessels of the lower third of the vaginal wall partly drain into the anorectal lymph nodes via the anal channels and partly into the iliac and hypogastric nodes. The upper two-third of the vaginal wall and the cervix primarily drain into the pelvic and peri-rectal lymph nodes. It should also be noted that the lymphatic disposi-tion of the genitoanorectal regions is subjected to considerable individual variations. The importance of the lymphatic drainage lies in locating the seat of infection.

MALE GENITAL ORGANS

The sagittal section of the male genital organs is shown in Figure 3.3.

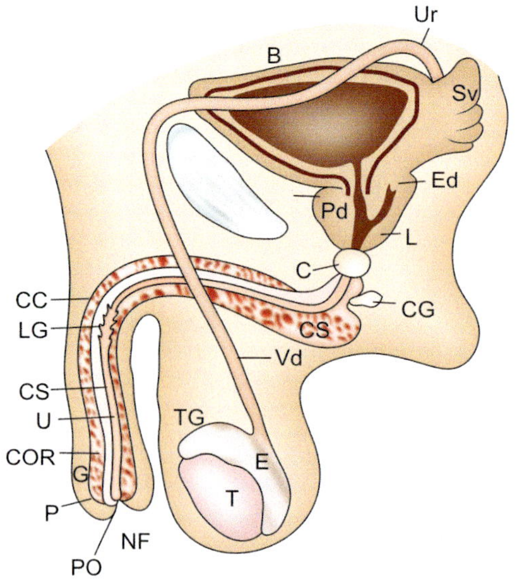

Fig. 3.3: Male genital organs. Sagittal section. **PO** preputial orifice; **P** prepuce; **NF** navicular fossa; **G** glans penis: **TG** Tyson's gland; **COR** coronal sulcus; **U** urethra; **CS** corpus spongiosum; **LG** Littre's gland; **CC** corpora cavernosa; **CG** Cowper's gland; **C** compressor urethrae; **P** prostate gland; **Pd** prostatic duct; **Ed** ejaculatory duct; **Sv** seminal vesicle; **Ur** ureter: **B** bladder; **T** testis; **E** epididymis; Vd vas deferens

Penis

It comprises a root and a free pendulous shaft. The root of the penis consists of three masses of erectile tissue lying in the urogenital triangle, which extends forward to form the shaft of the penis. The ventral portion of which is formed by corpus spongiosum and dorsally, it is covered by two corpora cavernosa. It is traversed by the urethra. It is the male organ of copulation.

Glans Penis

The corpus spongiosum expands to form-a conical enlargement, known as the glans penis. There is a groove demarcating the shaft of the penis from the glans known as the coronal sulcus. It contains numerous tiny glands, known as preputial glands, which secrete a bactericidal substance called smegma which has got a characteristic odour. It is covered by the free end of the corpora cavernosa. The skin covering the penis, folds upon itself at its terminal end to form the prepuce, which covers the glans. The internal mucosal layer of the prepuce which continues with that of the glans penis is a small median fold called the frenum of the prepuce. It is separated from the glans by preputial sac.

Prostate Gland

It is firm fibroglandulomuscular organ surrounding the commencement of the urethra which rests on the triangular ligament. It is conical in shape. It has a base, an apex, an anterior and posterior and two inferolateral surfaces formed by middle and two lateral lobes. The base is directed upward towards the neck of the bladder. The posterior surface is flattened from side to side, and slightly convex from above downwards. On the posterior surface there is a median groove which divides it into right and left lobes. Its apex is directed downwards and approximates with the fascia on the inner surface of the sphincter urethrae. The anterior surface is narrow and convex from side to side and extends from its apex to the base. The inferolateral surfaces are prominent and are related to anterior part of levator ani, surrounding the anal canal. The prostate is enclosed by a fibromuscular capsule. It shows branched glandular tissue, ending in acini, lined by columnar epithelium which is prone to infection, especially gonococci. The glands open into the prostatic urethra by numerous ducts. The ejaculatory ducts traverse through it and open at the floor of the prostatic urethra.

Urethra

It is a canal, the length of which is 20 cm. It consists of three parts; the prostatic, me mbranous and spongy urethra. The prostatic urethra is about 3 cm long. It starts from the neck of the bladder and extends downwards traversing the posterior lobe of the prostate up to its apex, where it continues with the membranous urethra. The latter is about 1.2 cm long and extends from the apex of the prostate to the bulb of the spongy urethra and it lies between the two layers of the triangular ligament. It is lined by transitional epithelium. The *Cowper's glands* lie on either side of it. They are two small rounded and somewhat lobulated bodies of yellow color. They lie above the bulb of the penis. They gradually diminish in size with advancing age. The excretory duct of each gland is nearly 3 cm long and opens into the floor of the spongy portion of the urethra. Each gland is made up of several lobules which are held together by a fibrous investment. The secretion of these glands is an additional constituent of the seminal fluid. The spongy urethra is about 15 cm long. It is a continuation of the membranous urethra and starts from the anterior surface of the triangular ligament and ends at the external urinary meatus passing through the corpus spongiosum. Distal to the membranous urethra it forms a dilated portion-the bulb, into which the ducts of the *Cowper's glands* open. Proximal to its terminal end it dilates to form the fossa navicularis. Many small glands such as *Littre's glands,* periurethral glands and *Tyson's glands* open into the spongy urethra. It is lined by columnar epithelium all through except the fossa navicularis, which is lined by stratified squamous epithelium.

Testis

The testis is an oval organ with flattened sides. The left testis is slightly lower than its counterpart. Its dimensions are 4 cm by 2.5 cm. It is contained in a pendulous scrotal sac made up of skin, fascia and dartos muscle. The testis is the reproductive gland of the male. The scrotum helps in maintaining the temperature below normal, for proper spermatogenesis.

Epididymis

It consists of a tortuous canal which is folded on itself. It is attached to the posterolateral surface of the testis. It consists of a body, head and tail. The tail of the epididymis continues to form the vas deferens. It traces its path and passes to the base of the prostate, where it is joined by the duct of the seminal vesicle, to form the common ejaculatory ducts.

Seminal Vesicles

These are sacculated pouches placed between the bladder and the rectum. Each seminal vesicle is pyramidal in shape and is 5 cm long, when it is coiled, and 10 to 15 cm long when it is distended. It is lined by columnar epithelium. It acts as a reservoir for the semi-nal fluid. As it is lined by columnar epithelium, it is prone to get infected in gonorrhea.

Lymphatic Drainage

The lymphatics of the glans penis, the prepuce, the shaft of the penis, the scrotal skin and the anterior part of the spongy urethra, primarily drain into the inguinal lymph glands. Ultimately they drain into the iliac glands. There is a free anastomosis of lymphatics of the scrotal skin, the penis, the spongy urethra and the anus. Hence, the involvement of one may affect the other. The lymphatics about the anus and to some extent the lower part (about two inches) of the rectum drain primarily into the inguinal lymph glands, but direct channels leading from the lymphatics about the anus, lymph nodes at the anorectal junction end in the sacral nodes along the posterior wall of the rectum. The lymphatics of the posterior urethra drain into the posterior pedicles of the prostate gland which empty into the rectal stalks and thence into rectal absorbent pedicles.

FURTHER READING

1. Johnson TB, Davies DV, Davis F. Gray's Anatomy (35 edn). London: Longman 1973.

Chapter 4

Gonorrhea

INTRODUCTION

Gonorrhea is an acute infection of the genitals, caused by *Neisseria gonorrhoeae,* characterized by pain, burning, frequency of micturition, and copious purulent discharge.

EPIDEMIOLOGY

Gonorrhea occurs all over the world and it tops the list of sexually transmitted diseases (STD) in India, and other developed and developing countries. It mainly affects the person of 20-40 years of age. The preponderance of gonorrhea over early syphilis and other venereal diseases has been attributed to several causes, namely a short incubation period during which infectious contacts need be traced. Further the reinfection is common in gonorrhea, for it does not leave any immunity at all. The latter becomes augmented when a single dose regime is followed for its treatment. Furthermore, invariably, the reservoir of infection is a woman, in whom gonorrhea has no symptoms, although to some extent it is true in men also. Nevertheless, they harbor the organisms and may unknowingly be the important source of infection, particularly if they belong to the permissive society. Other factors such as, lack of sex education, young age (teenage), civilization, urbanization, migrating laborers, immigrants, industrialization, increase in tourist traffic, affluence, prostitution and deteriorating areas or slums amongst socially disorganized group of low socio-economic status, may also play their role in its increase.

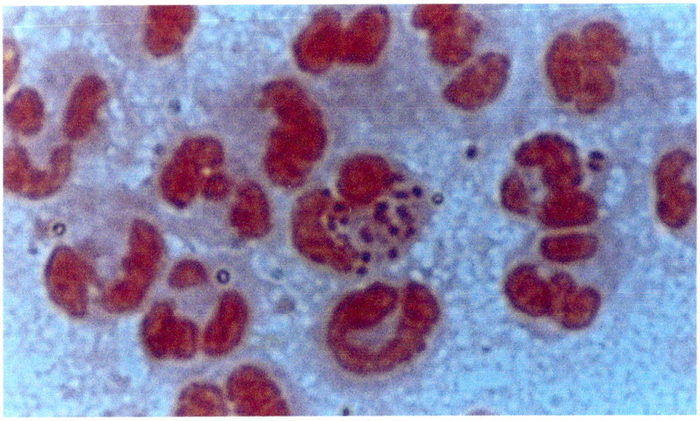

Fig. 4.1: *Neisseria gonorrhoeae.* Intra- and extracellular diplococci

ETIOLOGY

Gonorrhea is caused by *Neisseria gonorrhoeae.* They are gram-negative, oval or bean-shaped cocci of varying sizes. They are found in pairs with concavity facing each other. They are primarily intracellular, found in polymorphonuclear cells, but extracellular forms are also seen (Fig. 4.1).

It is a fastidious organism to grow *in vitro.* Various media namely

Thayer-Martin, Transgrow and Transport (Stuart's) media have been used. In these media nutrient agar is fortified by lysed whole blood or ascitic or hydrocele fluid. In addition the appropriate antibiotics are added to prevent or inhibit the overgrowth of other organisms. The culture media are incubated at 37°C in an atmosphere containing five to ten percent carbon dioxide for the optimal growth. The colonies of the organisms are characteristic. They usually appear after eighteen hours, but become prominent in the course of forty eight hours. They react positively to the oxidase test, turning pink to purple in color. They ferment glucose only.

PATHOGENESIS

The usual mode of transmission of gonococcal infection is by sexual intercourse, although the disease may be accidentally transmitted by other means (fomites), especially in children. The gonococci traverse along the urethral canal and succeed in penetrating the columnar epithelium of the mucous membrane, for which the organism has greater affinity. It excites an acute inflammatory reaction in the submucosa, resulting in the appearance of a variety of clinical features, depending upon the anatomical location of infection. Hence, in males in addition to urethra, *Littre's, Cowper's, Tyson's, periurethral* and *prostate glands, seminal vesicles and epididymis* are affected. In females, on the other hand, *urethra, Skene's* and *Bartholin's glands, cervix* and *fallopian tubes* may be involved. Besides, the spread of gonococci may occur through the blood (hematogenous), which may explain the occurrence of its metastatic manifestations.

INCUBATION PERIOD

This is variable. Usually it varies from two to ten days, with an average of five days. Most patients report in the course of 24-48 hours after the sexual exposure.

CLINICAL FEATURES

The clinical presentations and the course of gonorrhea depend upon the anatomy of the genital organs or affected parts. It is, therefore, different in males, females, and children.

ACUTE GONORRHEA IN MALES

The disease manifests as urethritis. It is characterized by pain, burning, and/or frequency of micturition. Hesitancy during micturition may at times be complained, following the preceding symptoms. Copious, thick yellow, purulent discharge per urethra (Fig. 4.2) is the classical presentation, especially when the urine is withheld for some period. At times the soiling of the undergarments may be complementary. In addition, constitutional symptoms namely mild fever, malaise, dizziness, and headache may be associated complaints (Table 4.1).

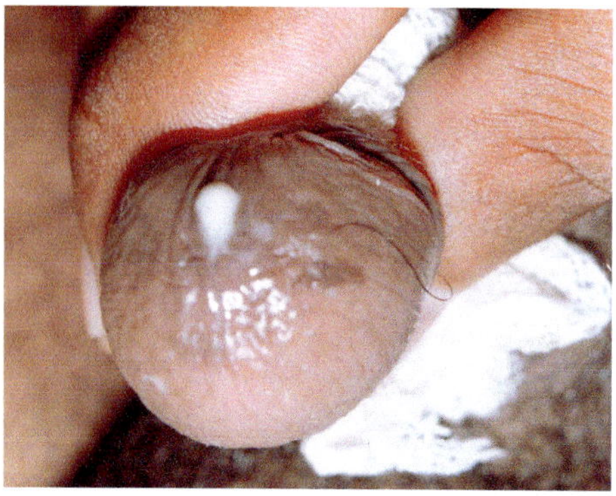

Fig. 4.2: Gonorrhea. A bead of pus at the external urinary meatus

The examination of the genitals reveals the presence of a thick, yellow, purulent discharge at the external urinary meatus. The urinary meatus is swollen, erythematous and tender. The palpation of the penile urethra elicits tenderness all along the penis. The enlargement and tenderness of the inguinal lymph nodes are sometimes observed. The anatomical localization of the infection is demonstrated by performing the two-glass test.

Two-glass test: Here the patient is instructed to void urine in two glasses one after another; haziness in the first glass suggests involvement of the anterior urethra, while haziness in both the glasses indicates spread of the disease to the posterior urethra. The presence of mucus threads in the urine denotes the involvement of the glands of urethra.

Urethritis may occasionally be asymptomatic, detected accidentally, while investigating the consort for the evidence of gonorrhea.

COMPLICATIONS OF GONORRHEA

The *Neisseria gonorrheae* may involve the adnexa of the genitourinary tract giving rise to acute complications, which may leave behind certain sequelae, and may result in metastatic manifestations due to probable hematogenous spread of the organisms or their toxins.

Acute Complications in Males

Tysonitis

It is an acute infec-tion of the *Tyson's gland,* charac-terized by uni-or-bilateral pea-sized abscesses on the side of the frenum. It may rupture through an opening (Fig 4.3).

Balanitis

At times there may be an inflammation of the prepuce leading to the formation of thick purulent discharge from it. On removal of the discharge, a raw, erythematous area is seen under-neath. It may cause phimosis.

Paraurethral Ducts

These are usually affected in urethritis, The orifices of the paraurethral ducts are edematous and red, which can be seen by everting the external urinary meatus. Additionally, the purulent discharge can be seen at the orifices (Fig 4.4).

Littritis

It is an infection of Littre's glands in the form of tender, minute swellings gently palpated along the course of the urethra. They can be demonstrated by passing an urethral sound which is, however, contraindicated in acute urethritis.

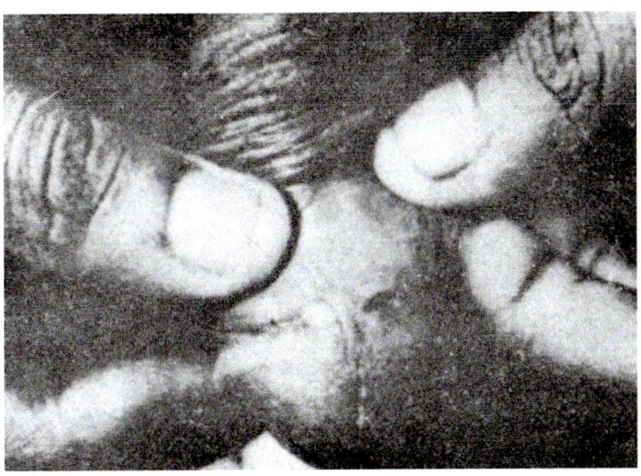

Fig. 4.3: Gonorrhea. Tysonitis—a pea sized abscess on the side of the frenum

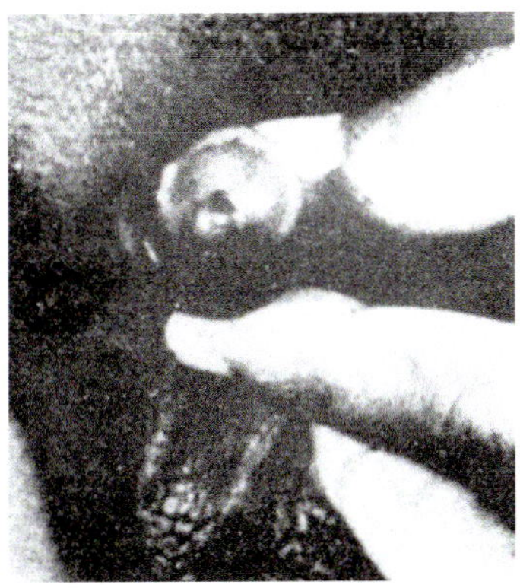

Fig. 4.4: Gonorrhea. Paraurethral abscess

Periurethral Abscess

It is either an infection of submucous coat of the urethra or extension of infection of the Littre's glands. The patient presents usually with a pain along the urethra or a periurethral swelling. It is tender and of varying sizes. It may fluctuate to open inside the urethra or on the shaft of the penis resulting in a sinus (Fig 4.5).

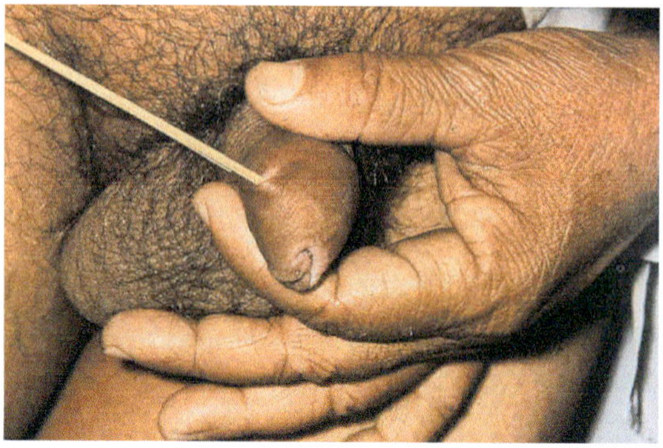

Fig. 4.5: Gonorrhea. Periurethral sinus

Cowperitis

It is an uncommon inflammation of *Cowper's* glands. The patient presents with a pain and heaviness in the perineum. It is apparent in the form of tender swelling, which may fluctuate and open in the perineum as a sinus, discharging purulent material.

Prostatitis

It is a rare, acute inflammation of the prostate gland, which takes place sometimes when the disease spreads to the posterior part of the urethra. The symptoms may be mild to severe from difficulty in passing urine to retention of urine. Pain while defecation and systemic complaints such as malaise and fever may be recorded.

Per rectum examination done gently, may show a large, tense and/or fluctuating swelling. The swelling may rupture into the urethra or occasionally into the rectum.

Seminal Vesiculitis

This is usually associated with prostatitis and the symptoms and signs are similar to that of prostatitis. Hematoma is noted sometimes, whenever the inflammation is severe.

Epididymitis

This complication is very rarely seen these days. The infection usually takes place because of retrograde passage of the infected urine. The condition is usually unilateral. Dragging to severe pain associated with systemic symptoms such as malaise and fever are the early symptoms. Initially, the lower end of the epididymis, but later whole of the epididymis is involved characterized by swelling and tenderness (Fig. 4.6). Secondary hydrocele is a common sequela. Sometimes the condition may lead to suppuration and may discharge pus through a sinus.

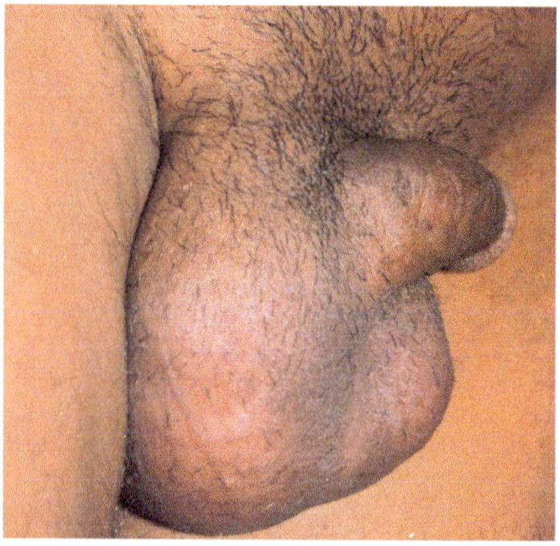

Fig. 4.6: Gonorrhea. Epididymoorchitis

Sequelae

The inflammation of some of the glands such as *Littre's, Cowper's, prostate,* and *epididymis* may continue to remain if prompt and proper treatment is not given to the patient, giving rise to chronic inflammation of these glands.

Strictures

If the submucosal tissue is severely involved in the acute stage, it heals up by the formation of fibrous tissue leading to strictures. Fortunately, this complication is only occasionally seen these days.

ACUTE GONORRHEA IN FEMALES

The disease is mostly asymptomatic or may have trivial symptoms, which may not attract the attention of the patient. It is, however, suspected in such females whenever their consorts apply for treatment.

In some patients it may manifest as acute urethritis. It is marked by pain, burning and/or frequency of micturition. Copious, thick, yellow, purulent discharge per urethra or per vagina may be present, especially when there is an associated trichomonal or candidal infection (Table 4.1).

The examination of the genitals may show erythematous, and/or edematous external urinary meatus. Also a bead of pus may be noted on milking the urethra. Per speculum examination may show mucopurulent or purulent discharge, in the fornices as well as their edema, erythema, and erosions.

Acute Complications in Females

Skenitis

It is an inflammation of *Skene's glands* which are lying on either side of the female urethra. The patient may report with pain in the urethra. On examination, either small abscesses at the external urinary meatus or a bead of pus is seen at the orifice of the *Skene's duct* on mild pressure.

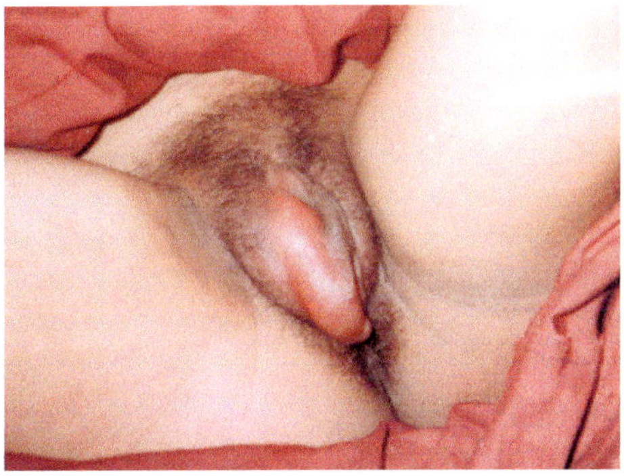

Fig. 4.7: Gonorrhea. Left Bartholin abscess

Bartholinitis

It is an extension of gonorrhea to *Bartholin's glands.* The reporting features are pain, heaviness of the genitals and difficulty in walking. The genital examination of the patient may show a swelling of varying size, it is tender and firm, located in the vestibule (Fig. 4.7). It may fluctuate to form an abscess which opens in the vestibule or on the skin surface.

Cystitis

The bladder may be infected in gonorrhea by extension of urethritis. It is the trigone of the bladder, which is affected. It is characterized by frequency of micturition.

Vulvitis

It is an uncommon involvement of the vulva by gonorrhea in adults. The vulvitis noted in these cases is usually because of the associated *Trichomonas vaginalis* or *Candida albicans* infection. Pain, erythema, edema of the vulva with thick purulent discharge is noted in such cases.

Proctitis

Gonococcal proctitis is a common complication due to the discharge trickling down to the rectum or at times, it may be due to rectal coitus with a patient of gonorrhea. Usually, this condition is asymptomatic, but sometimes burning and discharge may be the reporting complaints.

Acute Salpingitis

It occurs as a result of the spread of gonococci to the fallopian tubes. It is an acute episode characterized by constitutional symptoms such as fever, malaise and uni- or bilateral pain in the lower abdomen. The abdominal examination may reveal tenderness, guarding or swelling at *McBurney's point,* so that it may simulate acute appendicitis. If the symptoms are trivial it may progress to chronic salpingitis, revealed as a mass in the abdomen associated with backache of long duration. Occasionally, the disease is detected while investigating the patient for sterility.

METASTATIC MANIFESTATIONS

Arthritis

It is an unusual manifestation of gonorrhea. It may be due to hematogenous spread of *Neisseria gonorrhoeae.* It is characterized by acute symptoms such as fever, malaise, pain and swelling of the joints. It usually affects the knee and ankle joints. It is a purulent arthritis and may result in destruction of the cartilage leading to ankylosis. The gonococci can be demonstrated from the purulent discharge.

Gonococcal Septicemia

It is an acute condition, characterised by constitutional symptoms namely fever, malaise and dizziness. It may affect other organs resulting in acute myocarditis, pericarditis and meningitis.

ACUTE GONORRHEA IN CHILDREN

It is uncommon in children. The male children are rarely affected, while in female children it is infrequently seen. The infection is either acquired as a result of rape or by direct/indirect contact with infected persons. It manifests in children as *gonococcal ophthalmia* and *vulvovaginitis,* a pattern different from that in adults. Adnexa of the genitals are spared due to physiological variations in children.

Clinical Features

Vulvovaginitis

It may be asymptomatic or trivial or severe symptoms may be complained of by the child or the attendants. Whenever symptoms are present they are usually in the form of discharge, and burning sensation of the vulva. Sometimes burning and frequency of micturition are noted. In severe cases constitutional symptoms are also seen.

On examination, the vulva is erythematous, edematous with erosions, extending to involve the vagina. In addition, there is either watery, mucopurulent or thick purulent discharge. The rectum is similarly affected in some children. In male children the symptoms and signs are similar to that noted in adults.

Gonococcal Ophthalmia

Fortunately it is very uncommon these days. It affects usually infants in whom conjunctiva is amenable to Neisseria gonorrheae. It manifests as gonococcal conjunctivitis, recognised earlier as ophthalmia neonatorum-when the infection is acquired at the time of delivery, from the infected mother. The child presents with mucopurulent or purulent discharge, erythema and edema of the eyes. They may be associated with pain and photophobia. On opening the eyes after cleaning, the conjunctiva may show signs of acute conjunctivitis characterized by congestion of the palpebral and bulbar conjunctiva. In severe cases keratitis, ulcerations and perforations may be noted.

DIAGNOSIS OF GONORRHEA

In order to supplement and confirm the clinical diagnosis of gonorrhea in both males and females, the following tests are undertaken as office and/or laboratory procedures.

The specimens for the tests are collected by a platinum loop in the males from the urethra, while from the prostate it is collected from the prostatic massage only after four weeks in the follow-up period. Similarly, in females the specimens are taken from the cervix, the urethra and the rectum.

Smear Examinations

The smear is prepared, dried, heat fixed, and instantly stained with *Gram's stain.* The presence of intracellular gram-negative diplococci is strongly indicative of gonorrhea.

Fluorescent Antibody Test

It is of considerable use in cases where the gonococci are scanty. It is performed by adding globulin fractions extracted from antigonococcal rabbit serum, which is conjugated with *fluoresceine isothiocyanate* to heat-fixed smear from the discharge and incubated. The fluorescence under the ultraviolet light indicates the presence of gonococci.

Culture

The confirmation of instant smear diagnosis is, however, done by culturing the organisms on *Thayer-Martin* and *Transgrow media.* The inoculation of the discharge must be done directly on the medium and the same should be incubated immediately *(vide supra).* If it is not possible to do the same immediately, the material may be inoculated to the transport (Stuart's) mediat for subsequent inoculation in the regular media. Side by side the antibiotics sensitivity test is also performed.

Oxidase Reaction

The identification of the colonies of Neisseria is achieved by adding oxidase reagent which turns them pink to purple. Hence, its value is confined only to identify Neisseria colonies in mixed cultures.

Table 4.1: Acute gonorrhea

Males

1. Copious, thick yellow purulent discharge per urethra
2. Erythematous, swollen, tender external urinary meatus
3. Tenderness along the penile urethra
4. Occasional enlargement and tenderness of inguinal lymph nodes
5. Cloudy/hazy urine, either in one or both glasses in two glass test'
6. Tysonitis, balanitis, urethritis, periurethral abscess, cowperitis, litteritis, seminal vesiculitis, prostatitis, and epididymitis may complicate

Females

1. Signs and symptoms are trivial
2. Yellow, purulent bead of pus, at urethral orifice, after stripping (milking) the urethra
3. Reddened, edematous, external urinary meatus
4. Per speculum examination may reveal mucoid/mucopurutent/purulent cervical secretion
5. Reddened, edematous external os
6. Skenitis, bartholinitis, vulvitis, proctitis, and acute salpingitis (PID) may complicate

Fermentation Reaction

They are of considerable value in confirming the diagnosis, specially in medicolegal cases such as rape and divorce. A pure subculture of the organisms from the colonies is done on peptone-serum agar slopes, each containing one per cent of glucose, maltose, lactose and sucrose. The variations in fermentation of various sugars by different *Neisseriae* are given in Table 4.2.

Table 4.2: Sugar fermentation

Organisms	*Glucose*	*Maltose*	*Lactose*	*Sucrose*
N. gonorrhoeae	+	–	–	–
N. meningitidis	+	+	–	–
N. catarrhalis	–	–	–	–
N. phalyngis sicca	+	+	+	+

Complement-fixation Test

It is advocated as a diagnostic measure, but its value is limited only to academic pursuits.

Medicolegal Aspect

It is imperative to understand the medicolegal aspect of the diagnosis of gonorrhea. Many times the patient of gonorrhea is referred to a physician for opinion, especially where the legal proceedings in the case of rape or divorce are pending before the judicial court. The clinical diagnosis in these cases must invariably be confirmed by culture of the organisms, oxidase test and fermentation reactions.

TREATMENT

The treatment of gonorrhea consists of treating gonococcal urethritis and its complications, both in males and females. In order to ensure complete cure it is worthwhile to understand the principles of treatment. *Firstly,* the selection of the appropriate antibiotics to which the gonococci are sensitive is imperative. *Secondly,* by administering adequate dosage of the antibiotic, the high (vertical) level must be maintained at least for a period of 24 hours. The CDC recommendations for treatment of gonorrhea are summarized in Table 4.3.

Penicillin continues to be the mainstay in the therapy of gonorrhea in India and elsewhere, where PPNG is not a problem. Soluble penicillin-combination of crystalline and procaine penicillin (Cryst-4; Fortified procaine penicillin PPF-4) is preferred and administered intramuscularly in the recommended dosage of 4.8 mega units either in single or divided dosage. The effect of penicillin can further be enhanced by giving probenecid (Benemid)-a penicillin booster, orally in the dosage of 1 gm, a short-time before administering penicillin. Probenecid assists in maintaining the vertical level of penicillin, by impeding its excretion through the renal system.

Table 4.3: Gonorrhea treatment schedule

Infection	*Treatment of choice*	*Therapeutic alternatives to ceftriaxone*
1. Uncomplicated • Urethritis • Cervicitis • Proctitis • Pharyngitis (Patient > 8 years Exclude pregnancy)	250 mg of ceftriaxone I/M, single dose, followed by 100 mg of doxycycline, twice a day for 7 days	2 G of spectinomycin I/M, single dose For pharyngitis 9 tabs of sulfamethoxazole-trimethoprim (SMZ-TMP) (720-3600 mg) for 5 days or 500 mg of cipro-floxacin, single dose. Follow-up the treatment with doxycyline/ erythromycin
2. For patients < 8 years and pregnant woman	250 mg of ceftriaxone, I/M, single dose, Followed by 500 mg of erythromycin base, four times a day for 7 days.	

The alternative treatment, in such regions is:

- *Ampicillin (Eskaycillin; ampicillin):* It is a synthetic derivative of penicillin. It is as effective as penicillin. It is administered orally in a single dose of 3.5 gm, along with 1.0 or 2.0 gm. of probenecid (Benemid), which helps in keeping its blood level high. It is of no value in penicillin resistant gonococci and also in those who are sensitive to penicillin.
- *Amoxycillin (Hipen):* It is a bactericidal drug. Its bacterial spectrum *in vitro* is the same as for ampicillin. It is not effective against penicillinase producing organisms. It is given in the dosage of 3 gm, either as a single dose or in divided doses. It is effective in uncomplicated gonorrhea in males and females.
- *Cotrimoxazole (Septran; Bactrim):* It is yet another addition to the treatment of gonorrhea. The drug is available in the form of tablets, each tablet contains 400 mg of sulphame-thoxazole and 80 mg of trimethoprim. It is given orally either in a single dose comprising eight tablets or it is given in the dosage of four tablets at a time (stat) for three to four times, the interval between the doses being 12 hours. The cure rate of urethritis with cotrimoxazole is high, besides it does not mask concomitant syphilitic infection.
- *Tetracyclines:* They are also effective against the organisms. Any one of its derivatives such as oxytetracycline (Terramycin), chlortetracycline (Aureomycin) and tetracycline (Hostacycline) can be given orally in the recommended dose of 500 mg fourtimes a day up to a total dosage of 9.5 gm for 4-5 days. They are of limited value in pregnancy because of their side effects.
- *Erythromycin (Erythrocin; Althrocin):* It is also effective against the organism. It is administered orally in the dose of 1 gm initially, followed by 500 mg four times daily for a period of three to four days up to a total dosage of 10 gm. Erythromycin may be preferred because it is relatively free from side-effects.
- *Gentamicin sulphate (Garamycin; Genticyn):* It is also effective in its treatment. It is recommended in a single dose of 280 mg intramuscularly. Its tolerance is excellent and practically no side effects are observed.

FOLLOW-UP

Follow-up of the patients for a period of three months is imperative in order to ensure the complete cure of the condition and to prevent the spread of the infection. In the follow-up period the patient is advised to refrain from the sexual exposure. The patient is instructed to attend the clinic on the days as shown in Table 4.4. The history of exposure (during follow-up period), symptoms and clinical examination are recorded on each visit. Recording of the history of re-exposure is important to distinguish re-infection from relapse.

In males, the material for the smear and culture is obtained from the urethra and the prostate (prostatic massage), while in females it is obtained from the urethra, the cervix and the rectum. It is a practice to collect the material immediately after the menstrual period. Usually after adequate antibiotic therapy all the tests become negative by fourth to seventh day and continue to be negative throughout the follow-up period, unless there is re-infection or relapse or associated with postgonococcal urethritis (PGU). Post-gonococcal urethritis is diagnosed from the 7th to 14th day onwards, if pus count is over 30 per high power field in the *Gram's smear.*

In order to rule out concomitant syphilitic infection, as a rule, standard serological test (VDRL) should be done at the end of the first, second and third months.

In addition, recent World Health Organization (WHO) guidelines have been hailed as a break through for the treatment of Gonorrhoea and its subsequent complications (Table 4.5), which may ensure its cure.

Table 4.4: Follow-up

Days	*Symptoms*	*Signs*	*Two-glass test*	*Urine micro-scopic*	*Smears Gram's stain*	*Culture Stuart's, Thayer-Martin*	*VDRL*
1	Burning pain, frequency	Thick purulent discharge	Haziness in one/both	Numerous pus cells	Gonococci	+ve	Non-reactive
3	Mild	Mucopurulent	Haziness/ mucoid dis-charge	A few pus cells threads	Pus cells	– ve	—
7	Nil	Mild mucoid discharge	Mild haziness/ clear	A few pus cells	– ve	– ve	—
10 to 14	Nil	Nil	Clear	– ve	– ve	– ve	—
21							
28			Negative		Prostatic secretion a few pus cells		Non-reactive
2 months							
3 months							Non-reactive

Table 4.5: Gonorrhea treatment (Uncomplicated): WHO guidelines

- UNCOMPLICATED ANOGENITAL INFECTIONS
  Recommended regimen
  *Ciprofloxacin 500 mg orally, single dose
  Or
  Inj. Ceftriaxone 125 mg intramuscular, single dose
  Or
  Tab cefixime 400 mg, single dose
  Or
  Inj. Spectinomycin, intramuscularly, single dose
- DISSEMINATED GONOCOCCAL INFECTIONS
  Recommended regimen
  Inj. Ceftriaxone 1 gm by intramuscular or intravenous route, once daily for 7 days. Alternatively third generation cephalosporins may be used if ceftriaxone is not available, but more frequent administration will be needed.
  Or
  Spectinomycin 2 gm, intramuscularly, twice daily for 7 days. There is some data that spectinomycin may be effective for 3 days.
  For gonococcal meningitis and endocarditis same dose may be effective, but for endocarditis, the duration of therapy might be increased to 4 weeks.
- ADULT GONOCOCCAL CONJUNCTIVITIS
  Recommended regimen
  Inj, Ceftriaxone 125 mg, intramuscular, single dose
  Or
  Spectinomycin 250 mg, intramuscularly, single dose
  Or
  Ciprofloxacin 500 mg, single dose, orally
  This regimen is likely to be effective although there are no published data on its use in gonococcal ophthalmia.
  Alternative regimens where the recommended regimens not available
  Kanamycin 2 gm, intramuscularly as a single dose
- NEONATAL GONOCOCCAL CONJUNCTIVITIS
  Inj. Ceftriaxone 50 mg/kg, intramuscularly to a maximum dose of 125 mg
  Alternative regimens where ceftriaxone is not available

Contd.

Contd.

Kanmycin, 25 mg/kg, intramuscularly as a single dose to a maximum dose of 75 mg
Or
Spectinomycin, 25 mg/kg, intramuscularly as a single dose to a maximum dose of 75 mg
Single dose ceftriaxone and spectinomycin are effective and addition of tetracycline ointment is of no additional benefit.
Prophylaxis of gonococcal neonatal ophthalmia
Silver nitrate solution 1% in the infants eyes
Or
Tetracycline ointment 1% to the eyes of all infants at the time of delivery
Recommended regimens for infants born to mothers with gonococcal infections
Ceftriaxone, 50 mg/kg, intramuscularly, as a singlre dose upto a maximum dose of 125 mg
Alternative regimens where ceftriaxone is not available
Kanamycin 25 mg/kg, intramuscularly as a single dose upto a maximum dose of 75 mg
Or
Spectinomycin 25 mg/kg as a single dose, intramuscularly to a maximum dose of 75 mg

Test for cure: In men, the criteria for the cure of gonococcal infection lies in the absence of discharge, clear urine and negative urethral and prostatic smears and cultures. In women, it is based on negative smears and cultures taken from the urethra, the cervix and the rectum.

*Ciprofloxacin is contraindicated in pregnancy and is not recommended to be used in children and adolescents
There are variations in the anti-gonococcal activity of the quinolones and it is important to use the most active.

FURTHER READING

1. Anonymous. Neisseria gonorrhoeae and gonococcal infections. Report of WHO Scientific Group. World Health Organization, Technical Report Series No 616, Geneva: World Health Organization 1976;65-91.
2. Anonymous: Centres for disease control: Sexually transmitted diseases: Treatment guidelines. MMWR 1989;38:S8.
3. Cohen MS, Cannon JG. Human experimentation with Neisseria gonorrhoeae: progress and goals. J Infect Dis 1999;179:S375-9.
4. Darville T. Gonorrhea. Pediatr Rev 1999;20:125-8.
5. Easmon CSF. The changing pattern of antibiotic resistance of Neisseria gonorrhoeae (editorial). Genitourin Med 1990;66:55-6.
6. Ison CA, Dillon JA, Tapsall JW. The epidemiology of global antibiotic resistance among Neisseria gonorrhoeae and Haemophilus ducreyi. Lancet. 1998;351:8-11.
7. Judson FN. Gonorrhea. Med Clin North Am 1990;74:1353-66.
8. Patel K. Sexually transmitted diseases in adolescents: focus on gonorrhea, chlamydia, and trichomoniasis—issues and treatment guidelines. J Pediatr Health Care 1998;12:211-5.
9. Sehgal VN, Srivastava G: Gonorrhea and the story of resistant Neisseria gonorrhoeae. Int J Dermatol 1987;26: 206-14.

Chapter 5

Nongonococcal Urethritis

INTRODUCTION

Urethritis is an inflammatory response of the urethra to varied etiological agents, characterized by any or all of the following features.

- Urethral discharge
- Dysuria, Hesitancy and/or frequency
- Itch in the urethra
- Increased number of polymorphonuclear leukocytes in urethral secretion (4 or more per oil immersion field)

Urethritis is recognized as gonococcal and non-gonococcal urethritis (NGU). The latter is diagnosed on excluding *Neisseria gonorrhoeae* as the etiologic agent by smear and/or culture examination.

ETIOLOGY

Chlamydia trachomatis and *Ureaplasma urealyticum* are the main causes of NGU. Other microorganisms and non-sexually transmitted causes account for a small percentage. In the rest, the etiologic agent may not be identified.

Postgonococcal urethritis is diagnosed after adequate treatment of gonorrhea that eradicates *N. gonorrhoeae.* The other microorganisms may persist despite the treatment and the features of NGU are then unmasked.

The non-sexually transmitted causes may at times result in NGU. Thus, urethritis may be associated with urinary tract infection, urethral strictures, urethra valves, phimosis, and secondary to catheterization or instrumentation in the urethra.

Table 5.1: Etiology of sexually transmitted NGU

	Agents	*Percentage*
1.	*C. trahomatis*	30-50%
2.	*U. urealyticum*	20-40%
3.	Others	
	A. Bacteria	
	1. *Staphylococcus saprophyticus*	
	2. *Corynebacterium genitalum*	
	3. Anaerobic gram-negative rods	
	B. Yeast	
	1. *Candida albicans*	
	C. Parasites	
	1. *Trichomonas vaginalis*	
	D. Virus	
	1. *Herpes genitalis*	
4.	*Unknown*	20-30 %

CLINICAL FEATURES

NGU affects predominantly sexually active young individuals, in the age group of 15-29 years. The incubation period is 1-5 weeks, with a peak of 2-3 weeks. The classical symptoms include:

- Urethral discharge, which is usually mucoid/mucopurulent and scant. It may be noted only in the morning (morning gleet).
- Burning micturition. At times dysuria is mild or absent.
- Urethral itch.

The symptoms in NGU are mild and less florid than those in gonococcal urethritis. The latter is characterized by copious, yellowish-green, purulent discharge. Dysuria, frequency and hesitancy of micturition are marked. Genital examination is characterized by a slight grayish-white mucoid/ mucopurulent discharge or it may be clear fluid mixed with varying amounts of mucoid secretions. The discharge may not be obvious. In such cases, urethra needs to be stripped (milked) from base to the meatus 2 to 3 times. If the discharge fails to appear even after this maneuver, the patient is asked to report the next day after holding the urine overnight. Besides the discharge, the signs of meatitis may be visible, though, often it is mild or absent in NGU. The genitalia and the mucosae should be thoroughly examined for other lesions. The lymph nodes should be palpated.

DIAGNOSIS

The diagnosis of NGU is suspected on clinical signs and symptoms. However, a Gram stained smear is made to exclude the Gram-negative, intracellular reniform diplococci (*N. gonorrheae*), Besides, the smear is scanned at a magnification of X 100. The areas having polymorphonuclear leukocytes are then observed under the oil-immersion of the microscope. A mean of 4 or more PMNL per oil immersion field is diagnostic of urethritis. If the discharge is minimal or absent, a calcium alginate urethrogenital swab may be inserted 1-2 cm in the urethra to obtain the secretions. The PMNL may also be demonstrated in the urine. For this, the first 10-15 ml of urine is collected and centrifuged at 400 X for 10 min. All but 0.5 ml of the supernatant is decan-ted and the sediment resuspended in it. A smear is made from the sediment. After staining it is observed at a magnification of 400 X. Fifteen or more PMNL in 2 or more of the 5 high power fields is also suggestive of acute urethritis. Other investigations which can be undertaken are:

1. Gram-stain for *C. albicans* (*Staphylococcus*)
2. KOH smear for *C. albicans*
3. Swartzs Medrik stain for *C.albicans*
4. A fluorescein-conjugated monoclonal antibody immunofluorescent (Micro-Trak) test for *C. trachomatis*
5. An enzyme linked immunoassay for *C.trachomatis*
6. Culture of the urinary sediment on:
   - Thayer-Martin medium *(N. gonorrhoeae)*
   - Fienberg-Wittington/Bushby medium *(Trichomonas)*
   - Sabouraud's agar *(C. albicans)*
   - MacConkey's medium.

Treatment

Treatment of NGU is as outlined in Table 5.2.

Table 5.2: Treatment of NGU

Drugs	*Dosage*	*Status*
Tetracycline	500 mg, 4 times a day for 7 days Treat both partners.	Treatment of choice
Doxycycline	100 mg, 2 times a day for 7 days Treat both partners	Alternative to tetracycline
Erythromycin	500 mg, 4 times a day for 7 days Treat both partners	Useful for tetracycline resistant *U. urealyticum*
Amoxycillin	750 mg, three times a day for 7 days	Efficacy not well-evaluated
Trimethoprim/Sulfamethoxazole	160:800 mg, 2 times a day for 10 days	—do—

Recent World Health Organization (WHO) guidelines are a substantial to bring about a desired and effective change in the management (Table 5.3).

Table 5.3: *Chlamydia trachomatis* infections treatment (Uncomplicated): WHO guidelines

Doxycycline 100 mg, twice daily, orally for 7 days
Or
Azithromycin 1 gm as a single dose
Alternative regimens
Amoxycillin, 500 mg, orally three times a day for 7 days
Or
Erythromycin 500 mg, orally four times a day for 7 days
Or
Ofloxacin, 300 mg orally twice a day for 7 days
Or
Tetracycline 500 mg orally 4 times a day
Doxycycline and other tetracyclines are contraindicated in pregnancy
Current evidence indicates that extending the duration of treatment beyond 7 days does not offer any advantage
Erythromycin should not be taken on empty stomach
Azithromycin as 1 gm single dose is efficacious for chlamydial infections.
Chlamydial Infections during Pregnancy*
Recommended regimens
Erythromycin 500 mg, 4 times a day for 7 days
Or
Amoxycillin, 500 mg, orally three times a day for 7 days

Contd...

Contd...

Neonatal Clamydial Conjunctivitis**

All new borns with conjunctivitis should be treated for both N. gonorrheae and *Chlamydia trachomatis*, because of the possibility of mixwd infections.

Recommended regimen

Erythromycin 50 mg/kg in 4 divided doses for 14 days

Alternative regimen

Trimethoprim 40 mg with sulphamethoxazole 200 mg orally twice daily for 14 days

*Doxycycline and tetracycline are contraindicated in pregnancy

Preliminary data suggests that azithromycin is safe to be used in pregnancy, however the number of women in trials so far is too small to assess safety for use in pregnancy as adverse outcomes are likely to be undetected.

Erythromycin estolate is contraindicated during pregnancy due to drug related hepatotoxicity hence, erythromycin ethylsuccinate should be used instead.

**There is no evidence that additional therapy with topical agent provides further benefit. If inclusion conjunctivitis recurs after the therapy has been completed then erythromycin can be reinstituted for 2 weeks.

FURTHER READING

1. National guideline for the management of non-gonococcal urethritis. Clinical Effectiveness Group (Association of Genitourinary Medicine and the Medical Society for the Study of Venereal Diseases). Sex Transm Infect. 1999;75:S9-S12.
2. Robinson AJ, Ridgway GL: Concurrent gonococcal and chlamydial infection: how best to treat. Drugs 2000;59:801-13.
3. Taylor-Robinson D, Horner PJ. The role of mycoplasma genitalium in non-gonococcal urethritis. Sex Transm Infect 2001;77:229-31.

Chapter 6

Reiter's Disease

INTRODUCTION

Reiter's syndrome (RS) is a multisystem disease characterized by a triad of nongonococcal urethritis (NGU), conjunctivitis, and arthritis, in association with the mucocutaneous lesions of keratoderma blenorrhagica and balanitis circinata. However, largely the disease may not have all the well-known components and common presentation is the *forme fruste* of the complete syndrome. Inflammatory arthritis is the most frequent presenting feature of the triad. Accordingly, American Rheumatism Association (ARA) defined RS as "an episode of peripheral arthritis of more than one month's duration occurring in association with urethritis and/or cervicitis.

The disease occurs worldwide and appears 1 to 4 weeks after dysenteric/venereal infection. Majority of the patients are aged 16-35 years. It affects the males predominantly with male to female ratio of approximately 9:1 in the post-dysenteric variety and 99:1 in the post-urethritic variant.

Many infectious agents have been incriminated in the pathogenesis of this seronegative reactive arthritides.

These are shown in Table 6.1.

Table 6.1: Microorganisms causing Reiter's syndrome

Post-urethritic (Venereal) RS	Post-dysenteric RS
Chlamydia trachomatis	*Salmonella typhi murium*
Mycoplasma hominis	*Salmonella enteritidis*
Ureaplasma urealyticum	*Salmonella muenchen*
	Salmonella heidelberg
	Shigella flexneri
	Shigella dysenteriae
	Yersinia enterocolitica
	Yersinia pseudotuberculosis
	Campylobacter fetus ssp *Jejuni*

Affected individuals show a genetic predisposition to this reactive disorder as evidenced by the presence of HLA-B 27 in 60 to 70 percent of these individuals. The mechanism by which HLA-B27 confers the susceptibility to RS is debatable and yet to be established. However, different views are prevalent.

- The linkage disequilibrium hypothesis which postulates that on chromosome 6 is another gene that is responsible for the disease expression.
- HLA-B 27 gene is associated to this by linkage disequilibrium. B 27 acts as a marker for this disease susceptibility gene.
- HLA-B 27 genc modifies the immune response to infection HLA-B 27 provides a receptor site for the microbial pathogens.

- Cross-tolerance theory that hypothesises the cross-reactivity between B 27 and the microbial pathogens. An immune response is elicited and autoantibodies are formed. However, these show high affinity for microbial antigens and low affinity for the self-antigens.

The disease manifestations in HLA-B 27 positive and negative individuals are comparable. However, HLA-B 27 predisposes to chronicity, relapses, sacroiliitis and extra-articular manifestations.

CLINICAL FEATURES

Constitutional a symptoms like fever, malaise herald the onset of RS. Inflammatory arthritis is the most common presentation. It manifests as asymmetrical oligoarthritis that affects the joints of the lower limbs. Knee, ankle, midtarsal, metatarsophalangeal (MTP) or interphalangeal (IP) joints are often affected. Though any or all these joints may be affected together or sequentially over a period of 2 to 3 weeks, the manifestations are most florid in 2 to 3 of the affected joints. The joints are swollen and tender. The overlying skin may be erythematous. Tense effusions may develop.

Enthesopathy, (inflammation of the bone where ligaments, tendons and capsules attach, may cause severe pain. It affects the plantar fascia, insertion of Achilles tendon (lover's heel), chest wall and lower back. After the acute phase has subsided, the patient may continue to have persistent discomfort with interspersed exacerbations at varying intervals. These recurrent episodes also predominantly affect the ankles, midtarsal joints, metatarsophalangeal joints and the knees. However, at times elbows, wrist, sternocostal, costochondral, and temporomandibular joints may be involved. The signs and symptoms are less florid in recurrent episodes. Repeated exacerbation may ultimately result in periarticular fibrosis, contractures and bony ankylosis. Deformities may be a sequelae.

- Pes cavus
- Pes planus
- Subluxation of the metatarsophalangeal joints (Luanoi's deformity) (Fig. 6.1)
- Dorsiflexion at the metatarsophalangeal joints and hyperflexion at interphalangeal joints, (hammer toe deformity) subluxation at metacarpophalangeal joints with ulnar devialion (Fig. 6.2)

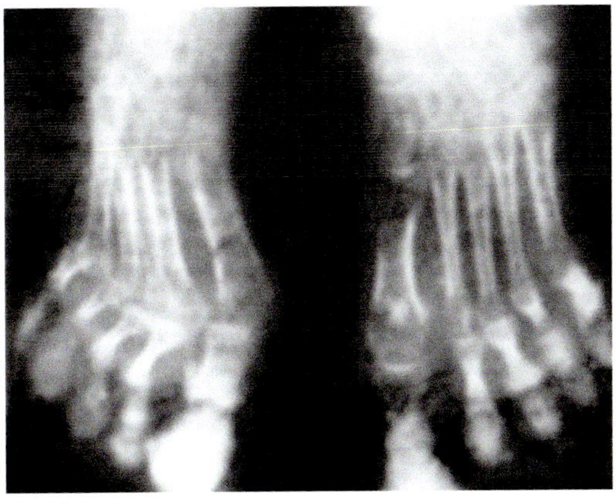

Fig. 6.1: Subluxation/dislocation of metatarso-phalangeal joint (Launois's deformity) of the feet with destruction of joints of the toes

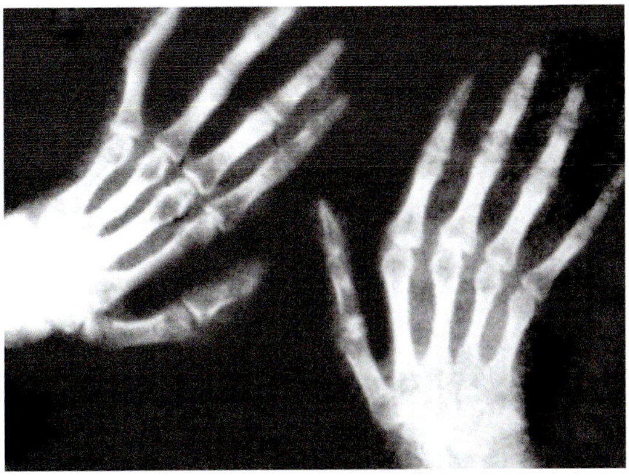

Fig. 6.2: Ulnar deviation and subluxation of metacarpophalangeal joints

Low backache, sacroiliitis, and spondylitis may also develop especially in recurrent episodes. The sacroiliitis resembles that in ankylosing spondylitis (AS). However, it is often unilateral and unlike AS, does not compromise chest expansion.

Genitourinary

They are often present in the complete syndrome as well as in the *forme fruste* of RS. However, at times they may be mild and missed by the patient. Urethritis is the most common genitourinary manifestation in either sex. In men, the infection may spread to involve the posterior urethra, urinary bladder, prostate, and epididymis. In women, the cervix, uterus, and fallopian tubes may also be affected.

Ocular

Conjunctivitis is the most common ocular manifestation. It is often bilateral and characteristically involves the tarsal conjunctivae of the lower eyelids at the lateral angles. At times mucopurulent discharge may be noted. However, in most cases it is mild and resolves spontaneously in a few days.

Anterior uveitis may develop during the recurrent episodes. It manifests as pain, redness, and photophobia and at times may be complicated by synechiae and secondary glaucoma. Associated sacroiliitis and HLA-B27 are markers for recurrent episodes of anterior uveitis.

Several other less common ocular lesions in RS are hypopyon, intra-ocular hemorrhage, keratitis, corneal ulceration, optic neuritis, and posterior uveitis.

Skin/Mucous Membrane

Keratoderma blenorrhagica, the characteristic cutaneous manifestation, affects 10-30 percent of patients of RS. Its incidence is higher in sexually acquired reactive arthritis. It affects the weight bearing areas of the palms and soles. However, scalp, trunk, and limbs may also be affected. It begins as discrete, waxy, yellowish brown vesiculopustules. These may coalesce to form well-circumscribed thick, hyperkeratotic crusted plaques (Figs 6.3A and B). Pustules may be interspersed among these plaques. The clinical appearance may be indistinguishable from pustular psoriasis.

The nails may also be affected and the changes may resemble those in psoriasis. The nails are dystrophic, thick, brittle, and discolored. Subungual hyperkeratosis and pustules may be present. At times the nail plate may show pitting. Ultimately onycholysis and nail shedding may occur.

Genital mucosa may be affected in 20 to 50 percent of cases. Circinate balanitis is pathognomonic. It begins as small vesicles on the coronal margin of the prepuce and adjacent glans. In non-circumcised males, these rupture to form painless shallow, red, moist, sharply demarcated serpiginous erosions. In circumcised males, these develop into dry, scaly hyperkeratotic plaques.

Shallow painless ulcers may be present on the buccal mucosa, tongue, palate, and fauces.

Cardiovascular system may at times be involved. Myocarditis, pericarditis, conduction defects, and aortic incompetence may result. Central nervous system may show features of meningo-encephalitis.

DIAGNOSIS

Reiter's syndrome should be suspected in any young adult with acute, asymmetrical oligoarthritis, affecting the joints of the lower limbs. The *forme fruste* of RS are encountered more commonly than

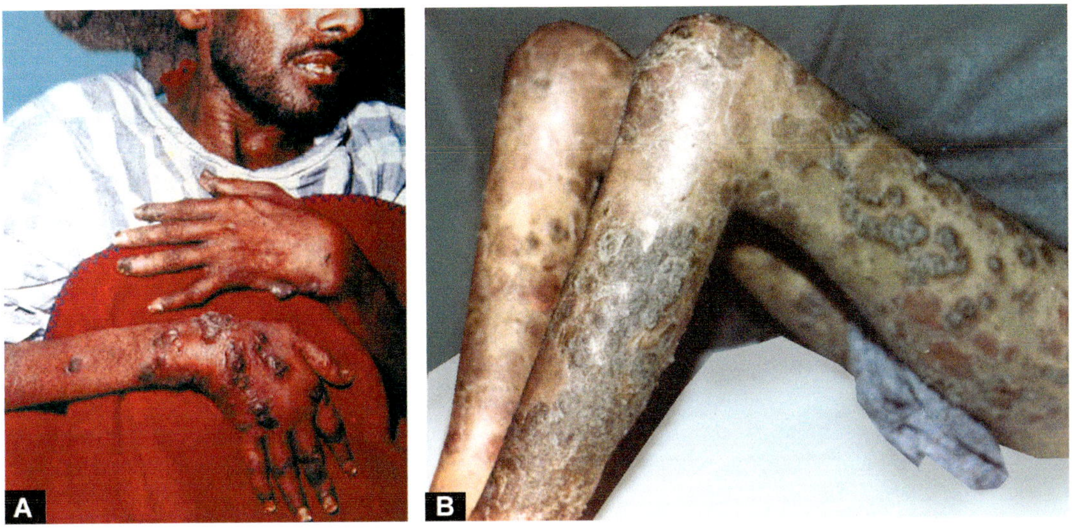

Figs 6.3A and B: Hyperkeratotic heaped up conical crusts on well-circumscribed plaques

the full triad. Accordingly history and signs and symptoms of urethritis/dysentery and/or eye affliction may or may not be forthcoming. The diagnosis has to be formed around the history and evolution of the disease and the cardinal clinical features. Laboratory investigations supplement but do not confirm the diagnosis.

Suggested Criteria for Reiter's Disease

- Typical acute arthritis
  1. Seronegative, asymmetrical
  2. Predominantly lower limb
  3. Heel pain, 'Sausage' toes
- Plus one or more of the following
  1. Urethritis
  2. Conjunctivitis
  3. Mucocutaneous disease (balanitis, keratoderma, oral ulceration)
  4. Preceding dysentery/non-specific urethritis.
- The other laboratory parameters that are revealed are:
  1. Normocytic normochromic anemia of chronic disease
  2. Polymorphonuclear leukocytosis
  3. Raised blood sedimentation rate
  4. Elevated C-reactive protein
  5. Negative rheumatoid factor
  6. Negative antinuclear antibodies
  7. Normal serum uric acid
  8. HLA-B27 positivity in 60 to 90 percent
  9. Synovial fluid aspirate may have PMN's in acute and lymphocytes in the chronic phase.
  10. Urethral/stool culture are often negative.

11. An endourethral swab may at times be positive for inclusion bodies
12. Skin biopsy shows features of parakeratosis, hyperkeratosis, acanthosis, and the pathognomonic spongiform macropustule in the upper/epidermis. These resemble the histopathological features of pustular psoriasis (Fig. 6.4)
13. Radiological examination reveals:
    A. *Peripheral joints*
       i. Predominant involvement of the ankle, midtarsal, *metatarso-phalangeal* and interphalangeal joints
       ii. Periarticular osteopenia in the acute phase followed by:
          - Periosteal reaction,
          - Proliferative new bone formation
          - Restoration of mineralization
       iii. Narrowing of the joint space and subluxations
       iv. Diffuse enthesitis producing osteoporosis/erosions during the acute phase followed by mineralization of erosions and fibers of attachment. This produces shaggy and whiskered pattern. Later resolution of inflammation by extensive fibrosis that may calcify/ossify to produce fluffy bony spurs (calcaneal and plantar).
    B. *Axial joints*
       i. Unilateral/asymmetrical sacroiliitis with features of focal erosion of cartilage, progressive joint space narrowing, reactive sclerosis, and incomplete fusion
       ii. Spondylitis, characterized by
          a. Large non-marginal syndesmophytes, occurring in skip fashion
          b. At times squaring of the lumbar vertebrae (Fig. 6.5).

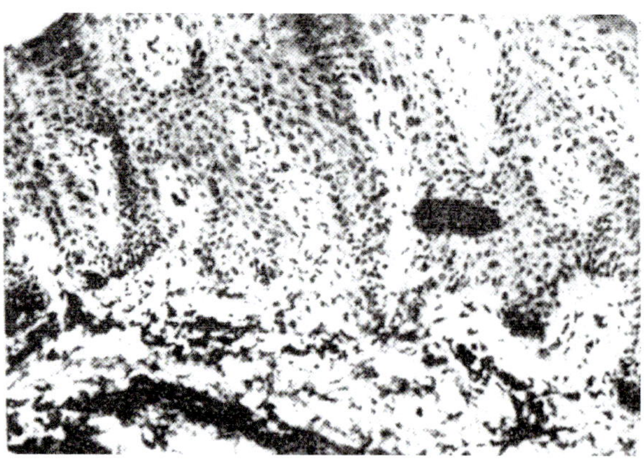

Fig. 6.4: A typical histopathology of Reiter's disease characterized by the presence of a large number of polymorphs and their condensation to form a pustule in the markedly hyperkeratotic and parakeratotic epidermis

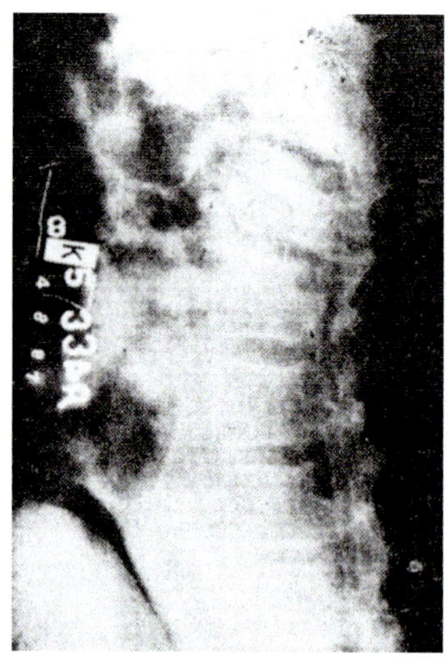

Fig. 6.5: Squaring of the lumbar vertebrae

Table 6.2: Treatment of Reiter's disease

Involvement	*Treatment of choice*	*Alternative*
1. Urethritis	Tetracycline/Erythromycin for 7-14 days	
2. Post-dysenteric	Fluoroquinolones	
3. Arthritis	Non-steroidal anti-inflammatory agents	In recatcitrant cases 1. Antimalarials 2. Systemic corticosteroids 3. Immuno-suppresants a. Methotrexate b. Azathioprine
4. Mucocutaneous	Topical corticosteroid	Ketoconazole retinoids

TREATMENT

It is outlined in Table 6.2.

FURTHER READING

1. Amor B. Reiter's syndrome. Diagnosis and clinical features. Rheum Dis Clin North Am 1998;24:677-95.
2. Bryant GA. Reiter's syndrome. Orthop Nurs 1998;17:57-62.
3. Leirisalo M, Skylr G, Kousa M, Voipio-Pulkki LM, Suoranta H, Nissilä M, et al. Follow-up study on patients with Reiter's disease and reactive arthritis, with special references to HLA-B27. Arthritis Rheum 1982;25: 249-59.
4. Parker CT, Thomas D. Reiter's syndrome and reactive arthritis. J Am Osteopath Asso 2000;100:101-4.
5. Sehgal VN, Koranne RV, Shyam Prashad AL. Unusal manifestations of Reiter's disease in a child. Dermatologica 1985;170:77-9.
6. Sehgal VN, Jain MK, Srivastava G, Saha MM. Reiter's disease: a radiological assessment of joints. J Dermatol (Tokyo) 1988;15:535-9.
7. Willkens RF, Arnett FC, Bitter T, Calin A, Fisher L, Ford DK, et al. Reiter's syndrome evaluation of preliminary criteria for definite disease. Arthritis Rheum 1981;24:844-9.

Chapter 7

Pelvic Inflammatory Diseases

INTRODUCTION

Pelvic inflammatory disease (PID) is an ascending infection of the female reproductive tract, characterized by the involvement of the uterus, fallopian tubes, and/or broad ligament. The infection may either be primary or secondary. The former may arise either.

- Spontaneously
- Acquired sexually

The latter may be the consequence of:

- Invasive intrauterine surgical procedures (dilatation and curettage, medical termination of pregnancy, hysterosalpingography or insertion of IUD).
- Parturition
- Abortion
- Caesarean section
- Hematogenous dissemination such as tuberculosis
- Extension from adjacent foci of inflammation such as appendicitis, ileitis, diverticulitis.

PREDISPOSING FACTOR

Several factors may predispose to PID:

- *Age*: PID affects young, sexually active women. Younger age is associated with lower protective antibody titres, larger zones of cervical ectopy that facilitates attachment of the pathogens, and greater permeability of the cervical mucus plug that allows the ascent of the microorganisms.
- *Sexual behavior*: Young age at first intercourse, high frequency of intercourse and numerous sexual partners (promiscuity) predispose to PID.
- *Contraceptive practices:* Intrauterine devices (IUD) are associated with an increased risk, while the use of oral contraceptives diminishes the risk of PID. Tubal sterilization may also reduce the risk of salpingitis.
- Gonococcal or chlamydial urethritis in the male sexual partner.
- Vaginal douching, the nature of douche solution, an douching technique may also flare up PID.

ETIOPATHOGENESIS

PID involves the ascent of infection from the lower genital tract to the fallopian tubes, with consequent invasion and development of salpingitis. Most cases are caused by *Neisseria gonorrhoeae* and/ or

Chlamydia trachomatis. Besides, numerous aerobic and an aerobic bacterial species that constitute the endogenous vaginal flora may also cause PID.

Anaerobic bacteria
- *Bacteroides spp*
- *Peptostreptococci*
- *Mobilincus spp*
- *Actinomycetes spp*

Facultative bacteria
- Enterobacteriaceae
- *Haemophilus influenzae*
- *Gardinella vaginalis*
- *Streptococcus* groups B and D

Mycoplasma
- *Mycoplasma hominis*
- *Ureaplasma urealyticum*

Several host factors tend to stop the ascent of these microorganism. These include:
- Unidirectional ciliary movement towards the uterus
- Flow of mucus in the fallopian tube towards the uterus
- Myometrial contractions

However, if the microorganisms succeed in reaching the adnexa, they might induce salpingitis. The pathogenesis of gonococcal PID differs from chlamydial PID. The human fallopian tube models are used to study the pathophysiology of gonococcal PID. When gonococci are incubated with fallopian tube explants, it is observed that:

- Gonococci attach to non-ciliated epithelial cells
- Endocytosis of the gonococci by the epithelial cells
- Intracellular movement of gonococci from the apex to the basal portion of the cell
- Exocytosis of gonococci into the subepithelium
- Ciliary stasis
- Cell death

The pathologic events are mediated by:

- Tumor necrosis factor liberated from tubal explant
- Complement component C5a

C. trachomatis also infects the columnar cells of fallopian tubes but produces little damage in tubal organ culture. Host response is more important in the pathogenesis of chlamydial PID.

- Attachment—it involves specific receptor-legend interaction
- Parasite endocytosis—the internalization into a phagosome
- Inclusion fusion—the *Chlamydia* containing phagosome is referred as an inclusion. Multiple inclusion in a cell may fuse
- Differentiation—within 8 hours, the elementary bodies (EB) differentiate into reticulate bodies (RB). These undergo division
- Reorganization—with 24-30 hours the RB reorganize into EB
- Release of thousands of infectious elementary bodies by either cell lysis or phagosome fusion with outer membrane.

The sequelae to chlamydial infection are mediated by the cellular immunity. The histologic changes reflect a predominant mononuclear response with some neutrophils.

CLINICAL FEATURES

The onset, severity, and the course of PID varies with the etiologic agent, the predisposing factors and the host response. The onset is acute often with constitutional symptoms in gonococcal PID. In Contrast, it is insidious and constitutional symptoms mild or absent in chlamydial PID.

- Abdominal pain is cardinal. It is usually dull and aching, Initially, it is localized to the mid-line due to affliction of the endometrium. As the infection ascends to the fallopian tubes, the pain shifts to affect the iliac fossae. Pelvic pain heralds the pelvic peritonitis. The pain becomes diffuse as the generalized peritonitis sets in.
- The patient may be febrile and have associated nausea and vomiting.
- Abnormal uterine bleeding, dysuria, hesitancy and frequency of micturition, anorectal pain, tenesmus, rectal discharge, and malodorous vaginal discharge may precede or accompany the abdominal pain.
- On palpation, the abdomen is tender. Rigidity, guarding and rebound tenderness characterize the peritonitis.
- Per speculum examination shows evidence of mucopurulent cervicitis.
- The movement of cervix elicits marked tenderness. This sign is called Chandelier's sign.
- Bimanual examination reveals uterine fundal tenderness due to endometritis and bilateral adnexal tenderness due to salpingitis. Adnexal swelling may also be present.

DIAGNOSIS

Its confirmation is hampered due to the lack of standardized criteria for interpreting clinical signs and symptoms, results of microbiological studies, histopathology, ultrasound and laparoscopy. The history and evolution of the symptoms namely onset with menses, presence of IUD, abnormal menstrual bleeding, exposure to a male with urethritis, abdominal pain, vaginal discharge, anorectal pain, tenesmus and discharge, hesitancy and frequency of micturition and the cardinal clinical features (vide supra) raise the suspicion of PID. However, it is necessary to undertake a battery of investigations to confirm the diagnosis and initiate therapy at the earliest so as to minimize the sequelae.

- Hemogram may reveal leukocytosis.
- Blood sedimentation rate may be elevated.
- Microscopic examination of a saline wet mount preparation of vaginal fluid often reveals more than one polymorphonuclear leukocyte 3 per vaginal epithelial cell.
- Gram staining of vaginal discharge may demonstrate gram-negative intracellular, reniform diplococci *(N. gonorrhoeae)*.
- A purulent fluid may be aspirated on culdocentesis, which will have polymorphonuclear leukocytes.
- Intravaginal ultrasonography has been explored as a non-invasive alternative to laparoscopy. However, it is not certain as to how advanced should the changes in the tubal morphology be, to be detected by intravaginal ultrasonography.
- Laparoscopy is the gold standard in the diagnosis of PID. It is mandatory when the diagnosis is in doubt. Laparoscopic criteria for the diagnosis of salpingitis include:
  - erythema of the fallopian tubes
  - edema of the fallopian tubes

– seropurulent exudate or fresh, easily lysed adhesions at the fimbriated end or on the serosal surface of the tubes.

These manifestations are more marked, tubes are not freely movable and patency uncertain in cases of moderate severity, Inflammatory mass may form in severe cases. Laparoscopy may also help in collecting the specimen from the fallopian tubes for culture and etiologic diagnosis.

- Endometrial biopsy may supplement the laparoscopic findings. It is useful in cases of silent PID, often caused by *Chlamydia trachomatis.*

Criteria for Diagnosis of Acute Pelvic Inflammatory Disease

All three of the following should be present:

1. Lower abdominal tenderness
2. Cervical motion tenderness
3. Adnexal tenderness (may be unilateral) plus

One of the following should be present:

1. Temperature >38°C
2. White blood cell count > 10,500/mm3
3. Purulent material obtained by culdocentesis
4. An inflammatory mass present on bimanual pelvic examination/sonography
5. Erythrocyte sedimentation rate > 15 mm/hr
6. Evidence of the presence of *N.gonorrheae* and/or *C. trachomatis* in the endocervix. Gram stain reveals gram-negative intracellular diplococci. Monoclonal antibody for *C. trachomatis*
7. Presence of >5 white blood cells per oil-immersion field on Gram stain of endocervical discharge.

It is important not only to make a diagnosis of PID, but also to identify the diagnostic markers that may identify the patient with a high-risk for sequelae like tubal scarring, infertility and ectopic pregnancy. The importance of such markers, if any, is further explicit in women with silent PID. The role of tumor associated trypsin inhibitor and tumor associated protein CA-125 as markers for subclinical tubal inflammation and as predictor for permanent tubal damage is being explored. Monitoring of lymphocytes for their *in vitro* response to tubal epithelial antigens may also aid in establishing the diagnosis.

DIFFERENTIAL DIAGNOSIS

Pelvic inflammatory disease needs to be differentiated from the following disorders.

Acute Appendicitis

It begins as periumbilical pain that may vary in severity from mild aching discomfort to severe. In a few hours, it shifts to and finally confine to the right iliac fossa. Anorexia is almost invariable. At times, vomiting and alteration in bowel habits may accompany the pain. Palpation of the abdomen reveals tenderness, rigidity and guarding in the right iliac fossa. Menstrual disturbance and discharge are conspicuously absent.

Ectopic Pregnancy

There is usually a history of missed menstrual cycle. After a short period of amenorrhea, the patient develops a severe lancinating pain in one of the iliac fossa. This is usually followed by profound shock, marked by pallor, low blood pressure, subnormal temperature and tachycardia. The lower abdomen is tender on palpation. Free blood in the peritoneal cavity is indicated by dullness in the flanks and intestinal distension in front. The patient has signs of shock. Vaginal examination may reveal an appendageal enlargement. However, it is better avoided as it may precipitate fresh bleeding.

Torsion of the Ovarian Cyst

It affects the small, mobile cysts. Initially it causes unilateral lower abdominal pain. As the venous return is obstructed, the tumor gets engorged with blood, the pain increases in severity. The patient becomes febrile and has tachycardia. Features of shock may develop. Nausea, vomiting and diarrhea may also develop.

Ruptured Ovarian Cyst

An ovarian cyst may rupture either spontaneously or following an abdominal trauma. Coitus may also precipitate its rupture. The patient notices a feeling of something giving away. This is followed by pain abdomen. Acute abdomen heralds the onset of peritoneal irritation.

Ovulation Pain

Mid-cycle pain (mittelschmerz) a common symptom affects women of the reproductive age group. It is characterized by pain in the hypogastrium and/or iliac fossa, and is experienced between 10th and 15th day. It varies in severity but usually subsides in 12-24 hours. The timing of the pain and its relationship to basal body temperature is cardinal.

Corpus Luteum Hematoma

It results from hemorrhage into and from corpus luteum. The patient experiences a sharp pain in the lower abdomen. The pain is usually followed by uterine bleeding, which results from the premature arrival of the menstrual period due to failure of corpus luteum. This condition may be misdiagnosed even at laparoscopy. It is essential to perform histopathologic study to confirm the diagnosis.

Diverticulitis

The patient presents with complaint of abdominal pain and altered bowel habits. Nausea and vomiting can occur and occasionally the patient may have abdominal distension, dysuria and/or rectal bleeding. Examination reveals abdominal tenderness, a painful mass and distension. The sigmoid colon is usually palpable. Tenderness is most marked in left lower quadrant and suprapubic region. Abdominal distension is generalized.

TREATMENT

The aim of treating PID is:

- To eliminate the infectious microorganisms
- To relieve the signs and symptoms
- To prevent tubal scarring and other sequelae and preserve the fertility.

Since therapy must often be initiated before microbial etiology is established, the treatment is usually empiric. Broad spectrum treatment is administered so as to be effective against poly microbial etiology of PID. The 1989 CDC treatment guidelines are summarized in Table 7.1. The outpatient regimen comprising ampicillin/amoxycillin with doxycycline/tetracycline and metronidazole, though discarded by CDC due to the emergence of penicillinase producing *N. gonorrhoeae* (PPNG), are still

Table 7.1: Management of pelvic inflammatory disease

	Indications	*Initial treatment*	*Maintenance*
Outpatient	1. Confirmed diagnosis 2. Mild to moderate illness 3. Reliable patient can follow the out patient regimen and can be called for follow up examination at 48 to 72 hours	Cefoxitin 2G, I/M + Probenecid IG, orally OR Cetriaxone 250 mg I/M	Doxycycline 100 mg, orally twice a day for 14 days OR Tetracyline, 500 mg, orally four times a day for 14 days
Inpatient	1. Uncertain diagnosis 2. Surgical emergencies cannot a day be ruled out 3. Severe PID 4. Suspected pelvic abscess 5. Patient in shock	**Regimen A** Doxycycline, 100 mg/IV twice + Cefoxitin 2G, IV, four times a day OR Cefotelan 2G, IV, twice a day For atleast 48 hours after cinical improvement	Doxycycline 100 mg, orally twice a day to complete 14 days
		Regimen B Clindamycin 900 mg IV thrice a day + Gentamicin, 20 mg/kg IV Stat and then 1.5 mg/kg IV every 8 hours for atleast 48 hours after clinical improvement.	Doxycycline 100 mg, orally twice a day to complete 14 days.

worth trying in count ries like India where the prevalence of PPNG is extremely low. Accordingly, it is imperative to update the treatment through recent recommendations of **Centre for Disease Control and Prevention (CDC)** appendix (10).

Besides, the specific therapy, the patient requires supportive therapy. These measures are guided by the clinical assessment and may include management of shock, intravenous fluids, Ryles tube aspiration, removal of the IUD, and care of the bowel and bladder.

Surgical intervention may be required if:

- Surgical emergencies such as appendicitis and ectopic pregnancy are suspected
- Rupture of tubo-ovarian abscess is imminent
- Pelvic abscess has formed
- Pyosalpinx
- Patient fails to respond to medical treatment

Laparotomy may be performed in these circumstances. However, if it reveals only PID, then any further surgical intervention is not undertaken. Specimen may be taken from the fallopian tubes for culture and sensitivity and the abdomen is closed.

FURTHER READING

1. Anonymous: Centre for Disease Control: Sexually Transmitted Diseases: Treatment Guidelines. MMWR 1989;38:S8.
2. Jacobson L, Westrom L. Objectivized diagnosis of acute pelvic inflammatory disease: Diagnostic and prognostic value of routine laparoscopy. Am J Obstet Gynecol 1969;105: 1088-98.
3. Korn AP. Pelvic inflammatory disease in women infected with HIV. AIDS patient care STDS 1998;12: 431-4.

4. Paavonen J. Pelvic inflammatory disease. From diagnosis to prevention. Dermatol Clin 1998;16:747-56.
5. Quentin R, Lansac J. Pelvic inflammatory disease: medical treatment. Eur J Obstet Gynecol Reprod Biol 2000;92:189-92.
6. Ross J: Pelvic Inflammatory Disease. BMJ 2001;322:658-9.
7. Sweet RL. Pelvic inflammatory diseases, and infertility in women. Infect Dis Clin North Am 1987;1:209.
8. Simms I, Stephenson JM: Pelvic inflammatory disease epidemiology: what do we know and what do we need to know? Sex Transm Infect 2000;76:80-7.
9. Westrom L. Pelvic inflammatory disease bacteriology and sequelae. Contraception 1987; 36:111-28.
10. Westrom L, Mardh PA. Acute pelvic inflammatory disease (PID). In Holmes KK, et al (Eds): Sexually Transmitted Diseases. New York: Mc Graw-Hill Information Centre Service Co 1990;593.

Chapter 8

Syphilis

INTRODUCTION

Syphilis is an infectious treponematoses caused by *Treponema pallidum,* transmitted usually by sexual intercourse, of great chronicity, systemic from the outset, affecting practically most of the organs of the body, marked by florid manifestations on the one hand and years of asymptomatic latency on the other, simulating many diseases in the field of medicine and curable to the point of presumptive cure.

EPIDEMIOLOGY

Syphilis occurs all over the world and it occupies the pride of place in sexually transmitted diseases. In India as well as in other developing countries the precise figures of its incidence are hard to get. Recently, there has been considerable decline in the late complications of syphilis, while early syphilis continues to manifest, applauding the triumph of specific antisyphilitic therapy.

It is, however, interesting to find the resurgence of sexually acquired syphilis amongst the younger generation in some developing countries, where endemic syphilis has been completely controlled. It is attributed to a considerable decline in immunity against treponemes. Other factors such as lack of sex education, young age (teenage), civilization, urbanization, migrating laborers, industrialization, increase in tourist traffic, affluence, and prostitution are responsible for perpetuating the disease incidence. Furthermore, deteriorating areas, slums among the socially disorganized groups belonging to the low socio-economic class may also play a complimentary role in its increase. It affects both men and women in the age group of 20-40 years.

ETIOLOGY

Treponema pallidum is the causative organism of syphilis. It was discovered in the Europe epidemic in 1905 by Schaudin and Hoffman. It is a slender, motile, brilliantly bright, spiral organism. Its length is 6-16 μ and width 0.13-2.3 μ. It has 6-12 spirals, each spiral is located at a distance of 1 μ. At its free pointed ends, tiny flagella like structures are seen. The organisms are recognized by their characteristic motility. It displays various movements namely slow undulating movement, corkscrew and to and fro movements.

It divides by binary fission, though its lifecycle is hardly evident. Its distinguishing features from the commensals are its slow clumsy movements, and regularly spaced spirals. It can only be seen by dark-ground, phase contrast and electron microscopy, because of its poor refractibility and slenderness. The organism can also be demonstrated in light microscope, when it is impregnated with silver.

The culture of the organisms has not yet been possible *in vitro.* It can, however, be propagated and kept viable in tissues like testes, scrotum and eyes of rabbits. The inoculation of the organism in apes, rabbits and hamsters results in manifestations similar to that in human beings. It has got a special predilection for the nervous system. It is unable to resist heat, drying, freezing and antiseptics like soap, glycerol and antibiotics.

Antigen Structure Immunity

No sufficient immunity is known to overcome the disease. Reinfection is, however, possible only when the earlier infection is adequately treated. The precise nature of the antibodies produced by *T. pallidum* is not sufficiently known. Nevertheless, it is capable of producing three types of antibodies in the serum, that is, non-specific antibody reagin detected by STS, specific antibodies detected by PTA and TPI tests, and group specific antibodies detected by the RPCF test.

PATHOGENESIS

The organisms invade the intact or abraded genital or oral mucous membranes through sexual intercourse or kissing. It may also be transmitted through blood transfusion, contaminated needles, and through the placenta *in utero*. It may be accidentally transmitted to doctors or nurses by indiscriminate handling of the infected lesions. It induces a local tissue reaction after a variable incubation period, determined by the size of the inoculum.

In the primary stage the perivascular lymphatics are infiltrated by lymphocytes and plasma cells. It affects the vessel walls resulting in necrosis due to endarteritis obliterans, thus forming a primary sore (Figs 8.1A and B). The organism invades the regional lymphatics inducing a similar tissue reaction (Fig. 8.1C). About eight weeks later the organisms disseminate to the various tissues, the reticuloendothelial system in particular, resulting in the secondary manifestations of the disease. The latter heal off by laying down of fibrous tissue to reappear again by the end of two years, if inadequate or no treatment is received. Later on the patient enters into the latent stage where there are no clinical manifestations of the disease. Three to five years after the secondary stage, the patient enters into the tertiary stage where the pathological lesion is a gumma involving the connective tissue and viscera. It is comprised of lymphocytes and plasma cells concentrated around the small blood vessels, giving the appearance of perivascular cuffing. The blood vessels show endarteritis obliterans resulting in necrosis with caseation. The epithelioid and giant cells are also seen. The fibroblasts are laid down at the periphery of lesion. The organisms may be scanty or absent due to massive destruction, representing a hypersensitivity reaction.

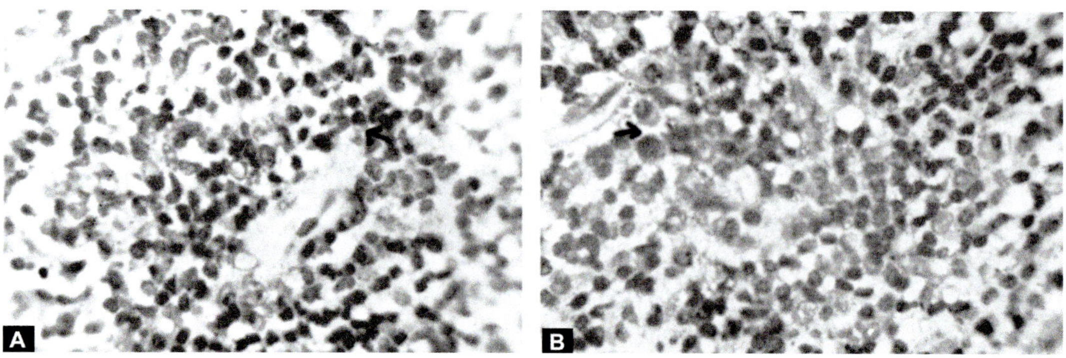

Figs 8.1A and B: Primary chancre. Plasma cell granuloma with endarteritis obliterans (H and E × 1000)

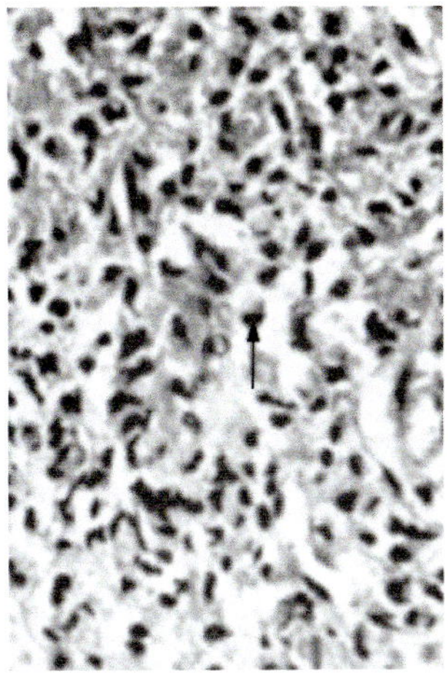

Fig. 8.1C: Secondary syphilis, condylomata lata. Plasma cell granuloma with endarteritis obliterans (H and E x 200)

CLASSIFICATION OF SYPHILIS

The clinical course of acquired syphilis may be divided into an early and late syphilis. The demarcation between the two is arbitrary and depends upon the duration of infections. In early syphilis the duration is two years. It, therefore, includes the primary and the secondary stage, relapses-clinical and/or serological and early latent. The sequences of events occurring after an interval of two years are covered under late syphilis. It, therefore, includes late latent, and tertiary syphilis consisting of gumma, neuro-and cardiovascular syphilis. In 20-30 percent of cases late complications may appear. The neurological complications may be asymptomatic, meningovascular or parenchymatous neurosyphilis. They usually appear 8-10 years after the inception of the disease, while cardio-vascular syphilis another significant late manifestation occurs after 10-18 years after primary infection. The sequence of events of the course of syphilis are shown (Fig. 8.2).

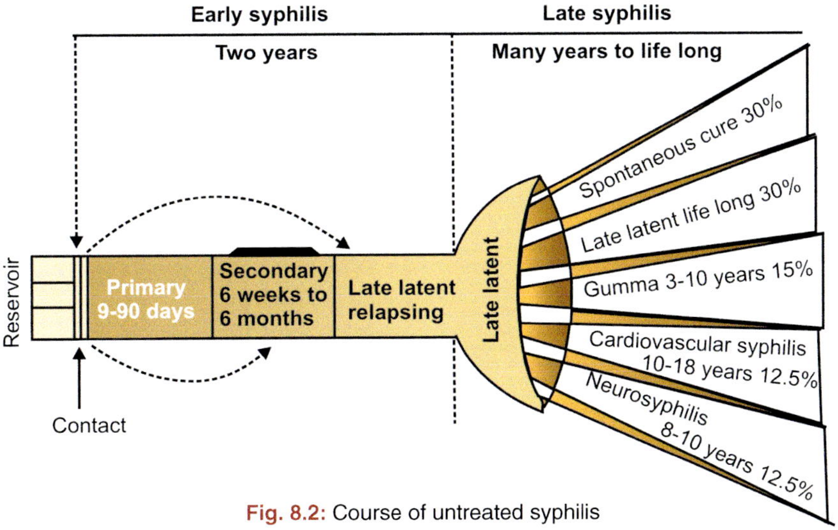

Fig. 8.2: Course of untreated syphilis

Early Syphilis

It comprises primary and secondary stages. Primary chancre characterizes this stage.

Incubation Period

It may have individual variations. Primary chancre usually appears after 10-90 days of sexual intercourse with an infected individual. Most patients report in the course of 15-21 days.

Clinical Features (Table 8.1)

Primary chancre: It starts as a painless, erythematous, indurated papule, which gets eroded in a short-time to form an ulcer. It is usually single. The ulcer is painless, clean, well-defined with a raw exuding surface. It is non-tender and markedly indurated, like a button glued to the skin or the mucous membrane (Fig. 8.3). Variations of the classical lesions may be seen in some patients. There is also a possibility that the presence of a primary chancre may be overlooked or concealed or that it may not develop *Syphilis d'emblee.*

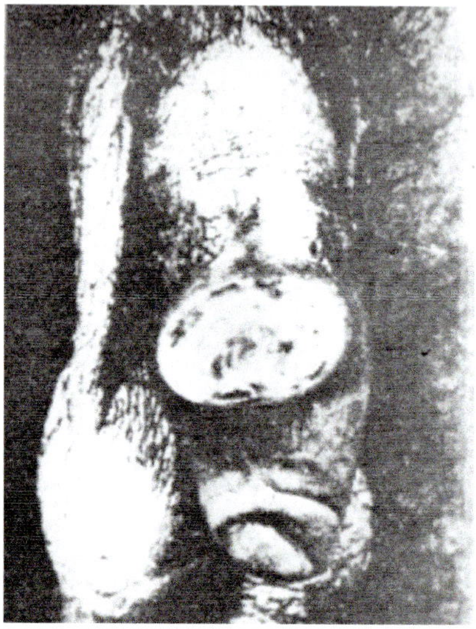

Fig. 8.3: Primary chancre like button glued to the skin

The ulcers may be multiple, showing a grayish-white *pedicle* on the surface. It may become painful and tender either because of secondary infection or because of concomitant infection with *Haemophilus ducreyi.* The latter is generally designated as mixed infection. The invasion of the ulcer with Vincent's organisms may result in gangrenous changes termed *Phagedena.*

The ulcer may heal spontaneously leaving behind tissue paper scar (Fig. 8.4).

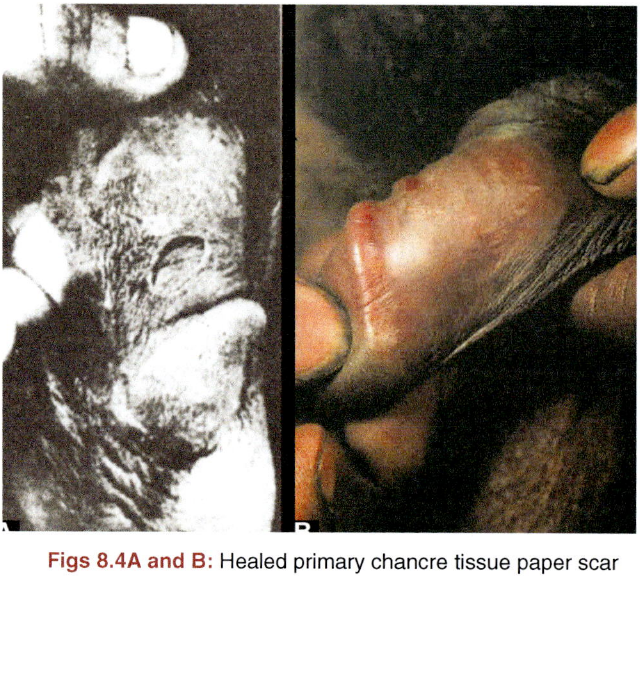

Figs 8.4A and B: Healed primary chancre tissue paper scar

Sites: In males, the primary chancre affects the coronal sulcus (Fig. 8.5) under surface of the prepuce (Fig. 8.6), the glans (Fig. 8.7), the preputial orifice (Fig. 8.8), shaft of the penis (Fig. 8.9), the scrotum, the external urinary meatus and the urethra (intraurethral). In females, it affects the labia majora (Fig. 8.10), the labia minora, the clitoris, the fourchette, the cervix, the vagina and mons veneris. The extragenital lesions are seen on the anus, the lips (Fig. 8.11), the breasts, the abdomen, and the thighs (Fig. 8.12). They also occur on the fingers amongst doctors and nurses.

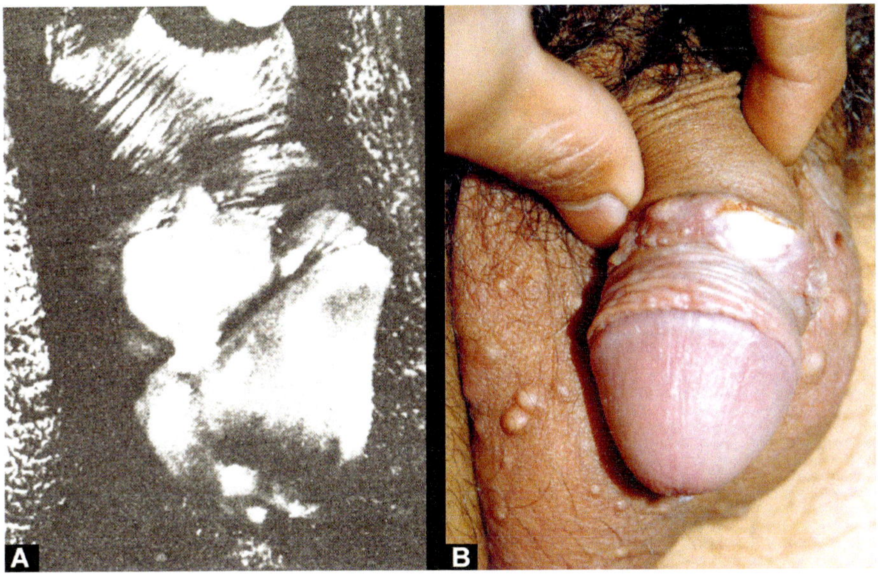

Figs 8.5A and B: Primary chancre affecting coronal sulcus

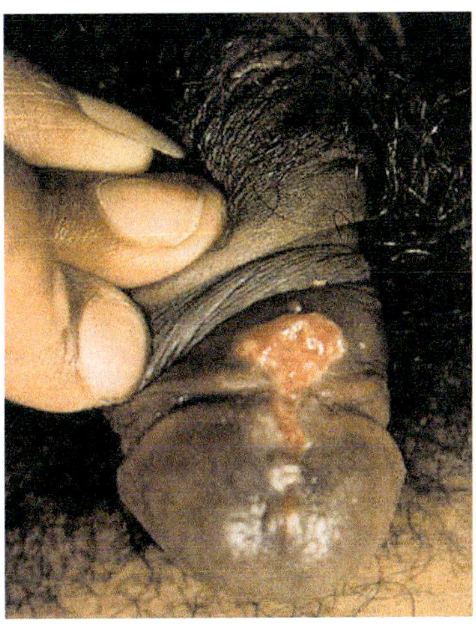

Fig. 8.6: Primary chancre on the under surface of the prepuce

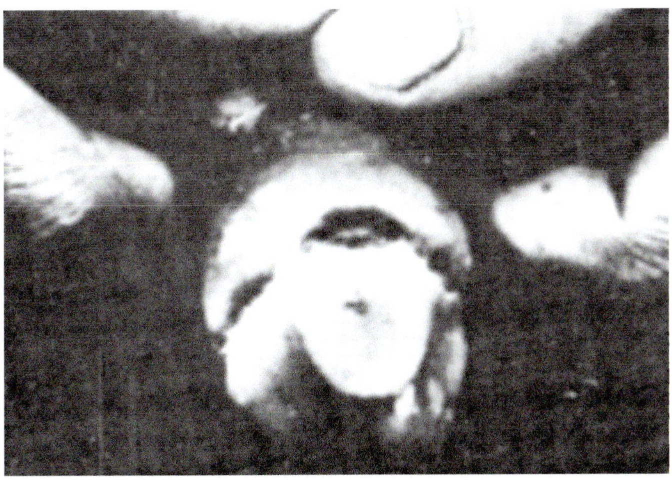

Fig. 8.7: Primary chancre on the glans penis

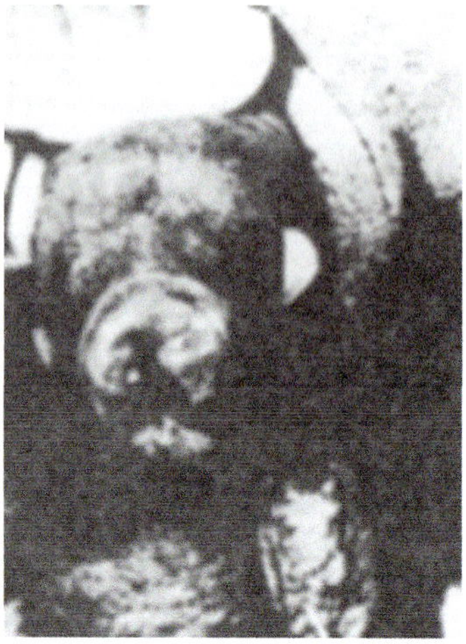

Fig. 8.8: Primary chancre on the preputial orifice

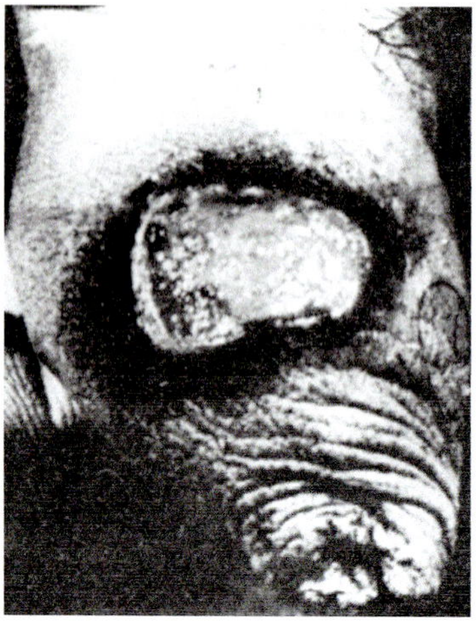

Fig. 8.9: Primary chancre on the shaft of the penis

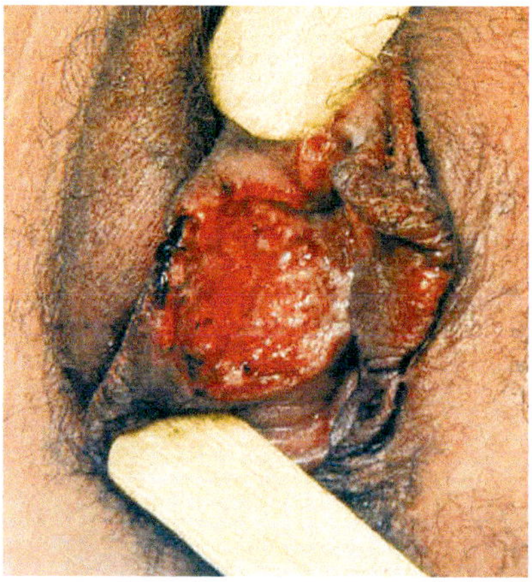

Fig. 8.10: Primary chancre on the labia majora

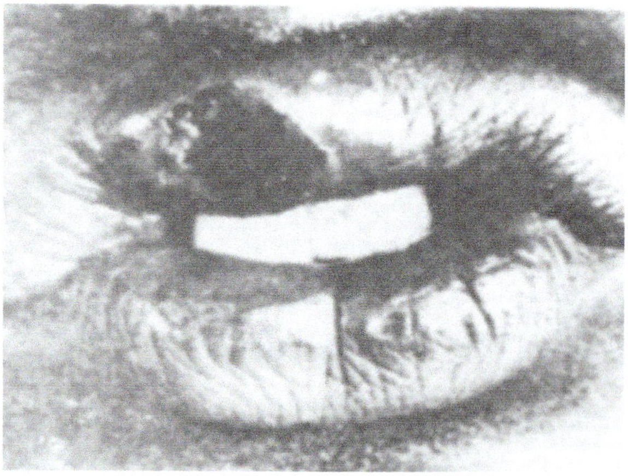

Fig. 8.11: Primary chancre on the upper lip

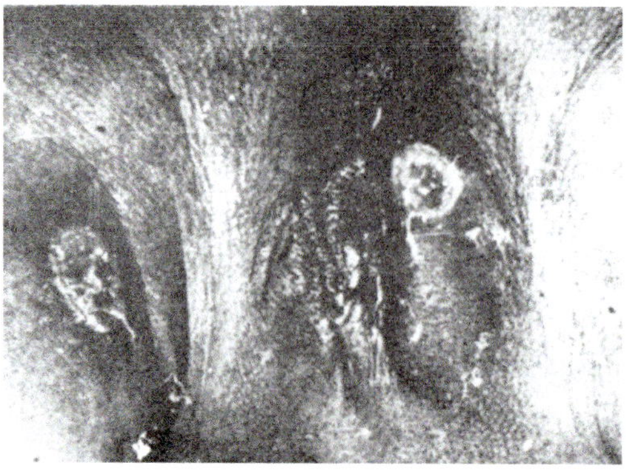

Fig. 8.12: Primary chancre on the labia majora and thighs

Lymphadenopathy: The inguinal lymph glands are invariably involved in the primary sore. They are recognized by their characteristic clinical features, that is they are multiple, non-tender, discrete, firm and mobile. They are usually bilateral in disposition. Similar regional glands may be noted in cases of extragenital chancres.

Diagnosis

In addition to the history and characteristic morphological features, the diagnosis is made by the demonstration of *T. pallidac* under the dark-ground microscope by regular wet preparations or by the direct fluorescent technique. The material for test is obtained both from the ulcer and the inguinal glands. The organism is recognized by its morphology, mobility and fluorescence. Standard serological tests should also be done, but their diagnostic value is limited, for the patient may report in the seronegative stage. Nevertheless, these tests are useful for follow-up. FTA-ABS and TPHA tests may be more useful than VDRL in early syphilis, for they are the earliest to become reactive. Other venereal and non-venereal ulcers on the genitals need be differentiated.

Secondary Syphilis

It is an indication of generalization of the infection, predominantly affecting the skin and the mucous membrane, characterized by polymorphous eruptions. The eruptions usually appear after an interval of 1-6 months after the appearance of the primary chancre.

Clinical Features

Usually the patient reports with constitutional symptoms like fever, malaise, bodyache, lacrimation and eruptions over the skin and the mucous membranes. Some patients may come with multiple swellings all over the body. The examination of the skin surface must be done in the day light which reveals lesions of different morphology. Their features may differ on the skin and the mucous membranes.

Skin: They are recognized by their characteristic clinical features, that is they are largely asymptomatic, generalized, reddish-brown in color and are of flexural disposition. The lesions are polymorphic, the predominance of one or the other type of lesions, determines the morphological description of the syphilitic rash *syphilids.*

Macular syphilids: The rash is classical. It is apparent over the skin surface in the form of reddish-brown, erythematous, macules of varying sizes and shapes, affecting mainly the front and back of the trunk and the extremities (Figs 8.13A and B). At places, they become indurated and raised to form *maculopapular syphilids.* The typical roseolar rash is seldom seen in Indian and other black races.

Papular syphilids: They are characterized by multiple, erythematous, indurated, papules varying from a pin-head to pea size, present both over the glabrous and the hairy skin (Fig. 8.14) in the latter the papules are found in association with the hair follicle, described as *follicular syphilids* (Fig. 8.15). They are distributed on the scalp and the beard area and may cause a patchy loss of hairs, termed as 'moth eaten' alopecia. Another classical lesion is the corona veneris, so termed when the follicular papules are distributed along the hair line of the forehead. Pruritus of a varying degree may be associated with these lesions. The papules may be arranged in different patterns, depending upon their arrangements, different names have been given. The papules when arranged in a ring-like fashion are *annular syphilids* (Fig. 8.16). A large central papule with small satellite papules arranged around it in groups are *corymbose syphilids.* At times the papulosquamous eruptions resembling psoriasis are described as *psoriasiform syphilids* (Figs 8.17A and B).

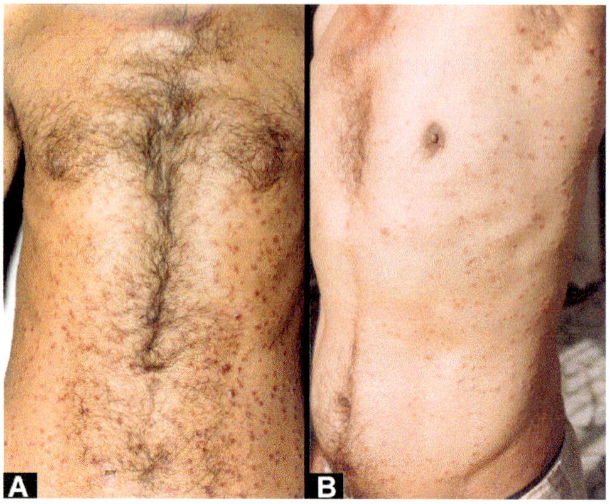

Figs 8.13A and B: Macular syphilids

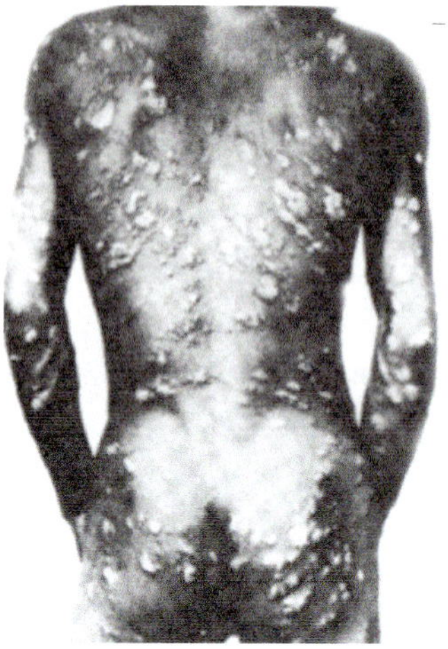

Fig. 8.14: Papular syphilids

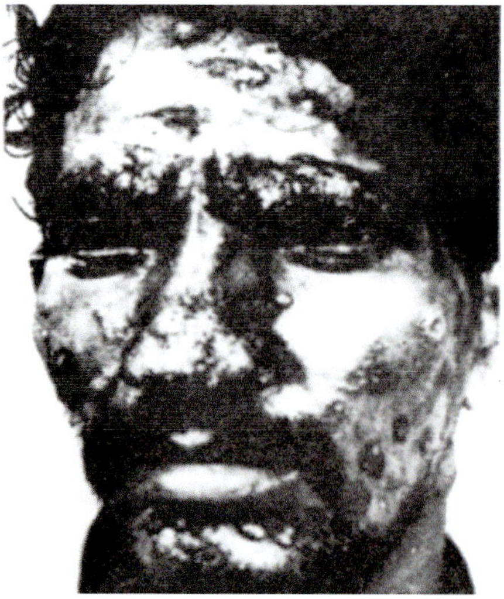

Fig. 8.15: Follicular syphilids

Fig. 8.16: Annular syphilids

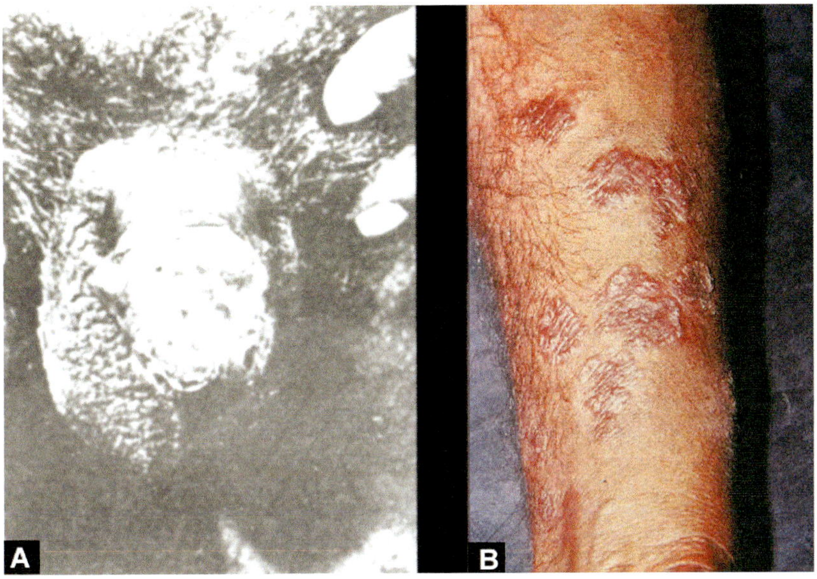

Figs 8.17A and B: Psoriasiform syphilids

Condylomata lata: They are the well-recognized lesions. They are broad-based, flat-topped, grayish-white, moist indurated, fleshy papules located in the body folds. They are commonly seen on the genitals (Fig. 8.18), the anus (Fig. 8.19), the axillae (Fig. 8 .20), the angle of mouth (Fig. 8.21), the groins, underneath the breast, and occasionally on the face (Fig. 8.22).

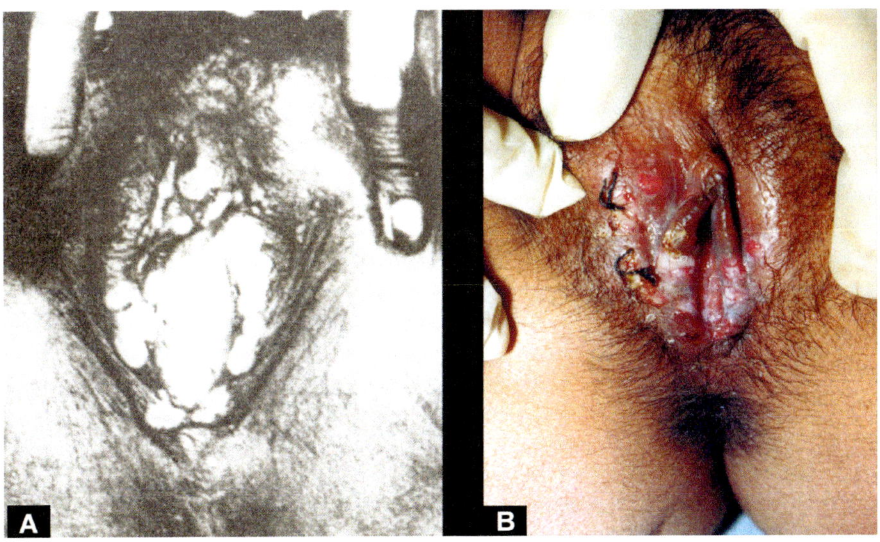

Figs 8.18A and B: Condylomata lata on female genitals

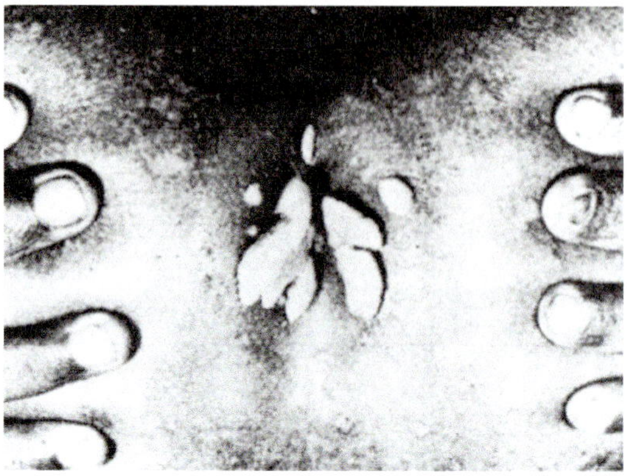

Fig. 8.19: Condylomata lata on the anus

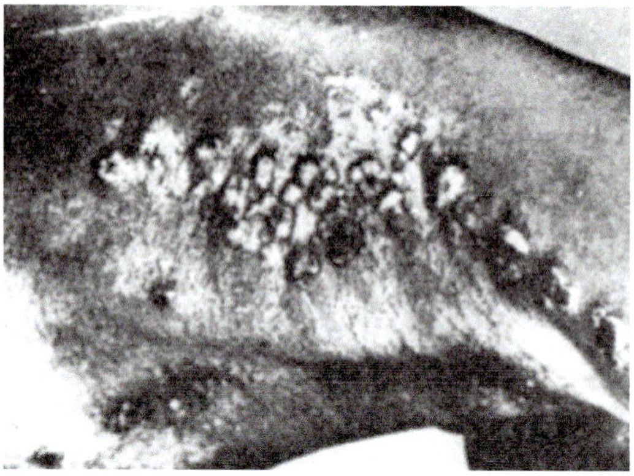

Fig. 8.20: Condylomata lata on the axilla

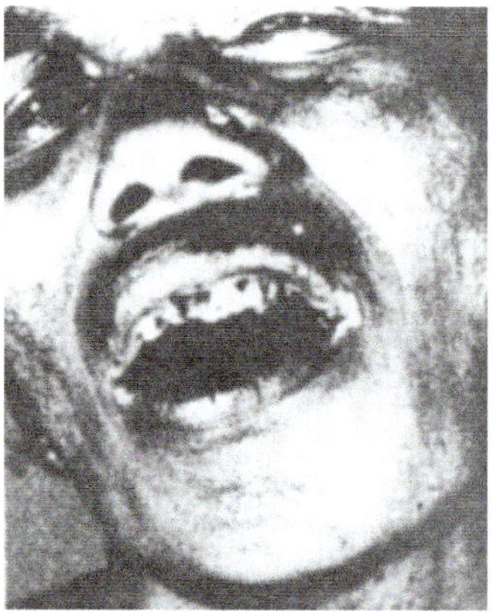

Fig. 8.21: Condylomata lata on the left angle of the mouth

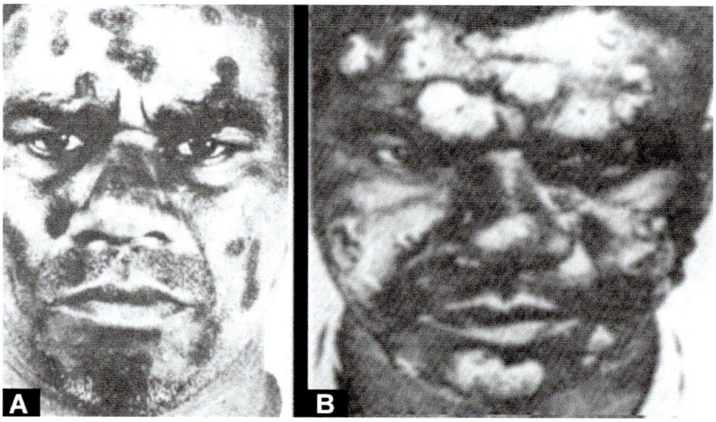

Figs 8.22A and B: Condylomata on the face before and after treatment (*Courtesy*: Sehgal et al. Brit J Vener Dis 1971;47:264)

Pustular syphilids: The skin surface may be studded with multiple pustules. They are because of necrosis of the papules due to endarteritis. Occasionally multiple, ulcerative, crusted lesions may appear over the extremities, face and trunk. These are termed as *syphilis maligna praecox* (Fig. 8.23).

Mucous membrane: Various morphological lesions over the oral mucous membrane may be seen. Mucous patches are the usual lesions, characterized by smooth, grayish-white erythematous lesions. These patches may get necrosed forming erosions or ulcerations. The ulcers may have an irregular or serpiginous outline simulating the track of a snail and are known as 'snail track' ulcers. The ulcers are primarily located on the palate and the cheek, while the mucous patches may be located on any part of the oral mucous membrane (Figs 6.24 and 6.25). Similar lesions may be seen on the mucous membrane of the genitalia.

Lymphadenopathy: In addition to the inguinal, the other lymph glands like the posterior cervical, axillary and supratrochlear may be involved. The clinical features of these glands are characteristic. They are multiple, non-tender, discrete, firm, and mobile.

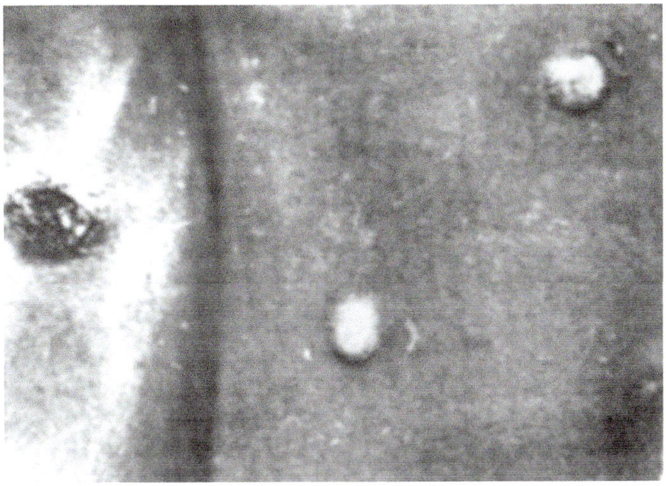

Fig. 8.23: Syphilis maligna praecox
(*Courtesy*: Sehgal and Rege, Brit Vener Dis 1974;50:237)

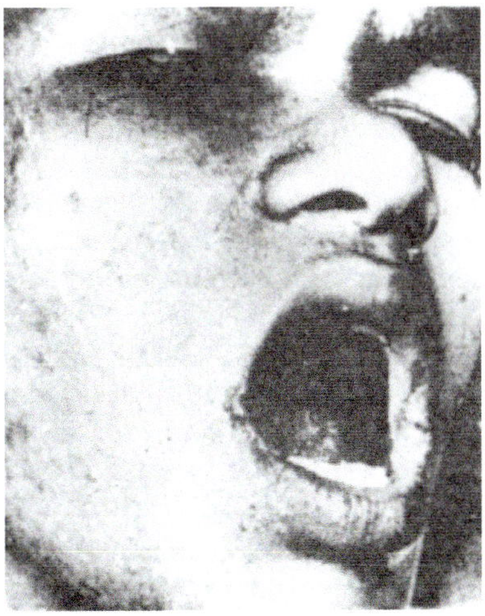

Fig. 8.24: Secondary syphilis: Mucous patches on the lips and tongue

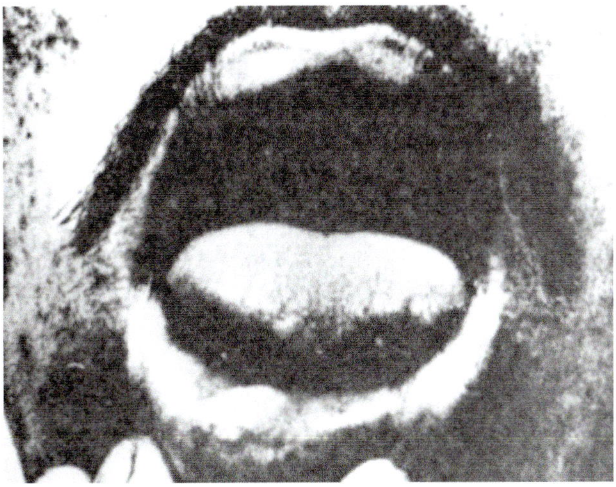

Fig. 8.25: Mucous patches on the tongue

Bones and joints: They form a part accompaniment of the diseases. The patient usually complains of a fleeting type of pain in the big joints. There may be swelling and/or effusion of the joints, and the movements of the joints may be considerably restricted . There may be involvement of the bones in the form of periostitis, with associated pain and tenderness.

Liver and spleen: The organs such as the liver and spleen may be affected causing hepatitis and splenitis, evident clinically in the form of enlargement of these organs. Occasionally the hepatitis may be associated with jaundice, specially in severe cases of secondary syphilis—*syphilis maligna praecox*.

Eyes: They may be involved in the form of iritis, characterized by pain, photophobia, lacrimation and circumcorneal congestion. In some it may cause choroidoretinitis. In others haziness of the anterior chamber with corneal opacities may occur. Initially one eye may be affected, followed by the other.

Central nervous system: The involvement of the central nervous system is rare in secondary syphilis, but when it occurs it is largely asymptomatic. Occasionally symptomatic neurosyphilis is also encountered.

In asymptomatic neurosyphilis certain cerebrospinal fluid (CSF) abnormalities are recorded without any apparent clinical features, whereas in symptomatic neurosyphilis certain symptoms and signs of meningeal involvement are noted in addition to the CSF findings. The patients may report with dizziness, headache, diminished vision and papilloedema pointing to the raised intracranial tension due to acute or subacute meningitis. Sometimes the cranial nerves may be implicated. The CSF examination, in these patients, reflects increase in globulin lymphocytes and a reactive serology.

Table 8.1: Clinical features of early syphilis

Primary chancre

1. A clean button-like, markedly indurated, non-tender, punched out ulcer, that oozes only serous exudate
2. Coronal sulcus, glans penis, prepuce, frenulum, shaft of the penis are predilection sites in men; Labia majora, labia minora, fourchette in women; Extra-genital chancre is uncommon
3. Characteristic rubbery, discrete, mobile, non-tender, and bilateral symmetrical lymphadenopathy
4. Self-limiting, usually heals with or without treatment.

Secondary syphilis (Syphilids)

1. Polymorphic, variegate, asymptomatic, bilateral, symmetric eruptions, predominantly of flexural disposition
2. Manifest as macules (roseolar rash), maculopapular, papular (follicular, annular, corymbose, psoriasiform syphilids, condylomata lata, pustular syphilids, and syphilis maligna precox
3. Buschkee-Olendorff sign, tenderness on pressing the papular syphilids, is cardinal
4. Vesicles are conspicuously absent
5. Grayish-white, smooth mucous patches, erosions, and 'snail track ulcers' on oral and genital mucosa
6. Generalized, discrete, rubbery, non-tender lymphadenopathy
7. Bones and joints, liver, spleen, and eyes may occasionally be affected

Diagnosis: It is made by the characteristic clinical presentation. It is confirmed by the demonstration of *T. pallidum* under dark-ground and fluorescent microscopy (Fig. 8.26). It is important to note that *T. pallida* can be easily demonstrated from the moist lesions of condylomata lata, mucous membrane, psoriasiform lesions and lymph glands. Furthermore, standard and specific serological tests are invariably reactive in high dilutions.

Differential diagnosis: Macular syphilids needs to be differentiated from drug eruption-history of drug consumption, the rashes and absence of lymphadenopathy are the clinical pointers. Similarly, exanthemata such as measles and rubella may have to be excluded by their morphological characteristics. Pityriasis rosea and versi color may also create diagnostic problems. The presence of a herald patch and the disposition of the other lesions along the body cleavages are helpful in the former, while in addition to the clinical features, the demonstration of fungi in ten percent potassium hydroxide will confirm the diagnosis of the latter.

Macular and nodular leprosy, an important entity in the tropics, and subtropics, may create confusion in the diagnosis of macular and papular syphilid. Leprosy is recognized by its presenting symptoms and signs. The finding of *Mycobacterium leprae* in the smear and histology is, however, diagnostic.

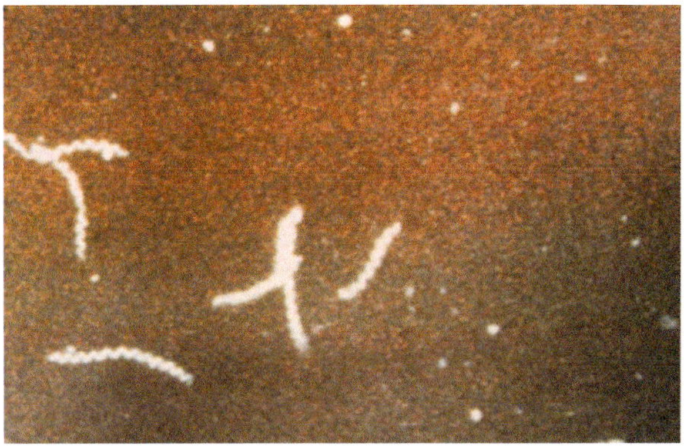

Fig. 8.26: Treponema pallida

In addition to *drug eruptions and pityriasis rosea: psoriasis, lichen planus* and *acne* may create some problems in papulosquamous syphilids. In psoriasis the distribution of the lesions and the Auspitz's sign, while in lichen planus itching and the flat-topped violaceous lesions, are the distinguishing features. In acne the history of seborrheic diathesis and distribution of eruptions at the seborrheic sites is helpful. In a doubtful situation, however, the diagnostic test for syphilis may clinch the issue. The situation may arise where the differentiation between condylomata lata and acuminata may be difficult. The former are broad-based and flat-topped in contrast to pedunculated and cauliflower-like lesions in the latter. Further confirmation is achieved by the reactive serology and the demonstration of *T. pallidum* in condylomata lata.

Pustular syphilids may resemble *pyoderma* and *exanthemata.* Clinical features and appropriate tests are helpful in their differentiation.

Angular stomatitis, *candidiasis* and *lichen planus* of the mucous membrane may create difficulty in the differential diagnosis of the mucous patch. *Aphthous stomatitis, tonsillitis* and *diphtheria* may have to be considered in the differential diagnosis of erosive/ulcerative mucous membrane lesions. Relevant laboratory investigations for each condition are required for confirming the diagnosis.

Course: In the course of time, with or without treatment the lesions of early syphilis heal up, leaving behind hypopigmented, atrophic scars. If the patient is untreated or inadequately treated then there is a likelihood of the patient going into latent syphilis and/or relapsing syphilis.

Relapsing Syphilis

Relapsing syphilis can occur during the first two years after acquiring the infection and is of two types—the clinical and the serological relapse. In the clinical relapse, lesions resembling secondary syphilis appear on the body, but they are usually few in number and less marked, than those seen in the earlier attacks. Mucous patches and condytomata lata are the usual lesions. Occasionally, a primary chancre may reappear on the original site and is known as *chancre redux or monorecidive.*

Serological relapse is indicated by the changing reactivity of the serum without any apparent clinical features. The non-reactive serum may turn reactive or already reactive serum may show a rising titer in the standard as well as specific serological tests. It may be heralded later by the manifest clinical signs.

Latent Syphilis

It is a situation characterized by reactive serology without any apparent clinical symptoms or signs. It is usually noted in the course of two years after the infection. It may be accidentally detected, while investigating the patients for the evidence of syphilis, antenatal check-up and in the blood donors. Specific-serological tests may be required to confirm latent syphilis. Later (after two years) it may continue as late latent syphilis.

Treatment

After the advent of penicillin, the earlier drugs, namely mercury and arsenic have become obsolete in the treatment of syphilis. The specific treponemicidal action of penicillin makes it the drug of choice for the treatment of syphilis. However, the maintenance of a sustained (horizontal) level of penicillin in the blood for at least a period of 10-15 days is an essential pre-requisite of the therapy. The usual effective level of penicillin is 0.03 unit/ml of blood. Furthermore, it is important to bear in mind that the patients must be treated adequately. It is, therefore, always safer to err on the higher side of the recommended dosage. It is, hence, a practice to administer penicillin parenterally.

Various preparations from the short-to the long-acting repository penicillins are now available. Any of them may be used for the purpose and the choice of preparation may be left with the treating physician. However, the long-acting repository penicillin is preferable, because it can maintain uninterrupted treponemicidal blood-tissue levels in contrast to the intermittent blood levels maintained by short-acting penicillin. Moreover, they minimize and/or eliminate the chances of defaulters.

Furthermore, long-acting repository penicillin, in particular, is ideal for single-dose mass therapy. The treatment schedule for early syphilis is shown in Table 8.2. The successful effect of penicillin treatment in the secondary syphilis is shown in Figures 8.22A and B.

Alternative Drugs

The administration of the alternative drugs is called for only when the patient is either sensitive to penicillin or when no clinical improvement is noticed after the adequate penicillin treatment. Tetracyclines and erythromycin are the alternative drugs. They have a definite treponemicidal action. Although these drugs have been used in the treatment of early syphilis since long, yet their precise impact on the subsequent course of syphilis needs be studied extensively.

Tetracyclines: Different derivatives of tetracycline such as oxytetracycline (Terramycin), chlortetracycline (Aureomycin), tetracycline hydrochloride (Hostacycline), demethylchlor-tetracycline (Ledermycin) and doxycycline (Duroxiline) may be used.

The latest CDC recommendations for treatment of syphilis are shown in Table 8.2.

Table 8.2: Syphilis treatment schedule

Stage	*Treatment of Choice*	*Alternatives for Penicillin Allergic Patients*
Early Syphilis a. Primary b. Secondary c. Early Latent	Benzathine penicillin, 2.4 million units, 1/M, single dose	100 mg of doxycycline, twice a day for 15 days Or 500 mg of tetracycline, four times a day for 15 days
* Late Latent Syphilis or Syphilis of Unknown Duration (excluding asymptomatic neurosyphilis)	Benzathine penicillin 2.4 million units, 1/M, weekly for 3 weeks (Total of 7.2 million units)	100 mg doxycycline, twice a day for 30 days Or 500 mg of tetracycline four times a day for 30 days
Tertiary Syphilis (Excluding neurosyphilis)	—Do—	—Do—

* Late syphilis: 1 year after infection.
Erythromycin: efficacy not well-documented.

Adverse Reactions

Immediate reaction: It occurs from a few seconds to 30 minutes after the administration of penicillin. There may be initial symptoms of weakness and malaise, accompanied by a skin rash. They may subside or progress to anaphylactic shock or shock may occur without prodromal symptoms.

Accelerated reaction: It occurs within 48 hours after penicillin administration. It is characterized by urticaria and/or angioneurotic edema.

Late allergic reactions: They occur usually after three days of administration of penicillin. They are characterized by serum sickness-like symptoms, cutaneous manifestations like urticaria, stiffness and pain in the joints, fever, and blood dyscrasias. Prompt and intensive treatment should be initiated for anaphylactic reactions, comprising 0.5 ml (1/1,000) adrenaline hydrochloride (epinephrine), followed by appropriate shock therapy. Otherwise corticosteroids, and antihistamines in the required dosage are useful in *accelerated* and late *allergic reactions.*

Jarisch-Herxheimer reaction: This reaction is believed to the due to endotoxins liberated from killed treponemes, following initial administration of the treponemicidal drugs, commonly due to penicillin. It results in both systemic disturbances and local reaction of the syphilitic lesions. The reaction is quite common in early syphilis. It usually appears within 24 hours of the administration of the first dose. The constitutional symptoms are marked by fever, bodyache, headache and lacrimation. Side by side there is an exacerbation of the existing lesions, i.e. edema develops in the primary chancre, the secondary syphilitic eruptions on the skin as well as mucous membrane become intense. Additionally there may be the appearance of new lesions. The reaction is favorable and transient and the patient may accordingly be informed before administering the therapy. Hence no treatment is generally indicated. Nevertheless, corticosteroids in the dosage of 15-20 mg daily and appropriate antihistamines may be useful.

Prophylactic Treatment

Penicillin as far as possible should not be used for the purpose. Prophylactic treatment should preferably be avoided.

Follow-up

The treatment is considered incomplete unless the patient is followed-up for a period of two years. In primary and secondary syphilis the clinical inspection and quantitative standard serological test should be performed, at monthly interval for a period of three months. Subsequently, at 6th, 9th, 12th, 18th and 24th month. Simultaneously at 12th and 24th month, it is worthwhile to perform CSF examination. Clinical relapse, serological relapse, a marked increase of titre, or evidence of syphilis in CSF requires immediate retreatment according to the recommended (vide supra) or enhanced schedule.

Late Syphilis

Late Latent Syphilis

It is the continuation of an early latent syphilis, that is two years after the infection. It may regress spontaneously or may continue for many years. Usually, it is accidentally detected during the antenatal check-up, in blood donors, immigrants, and at the birth of a syphilitic child. Apparently there are no symptoms and signs. The investigative evidence of affliction of any organ is lacking. Nevertheless, the standard and specific serological tests are reactive. It is however, imperative to investigate for the evidence of asymptomatic neurosyphilis before labeling the case as late latent syphilis.

Benign Tertiary Syphilis

Gummas characterize the benign tertiary syphilis. They usually appear three to ten years after the infection. They may affect the skin, mucous membrane, bones, joints and viscera.

Clinical Features

Skin: They may be nodular/noduloulcerative, papulosquamous/psoriasiform and subcutaneous.

Nodular/noduloulcerative: They are multiple, discrete, indurated, nontender and firm nodules, arranged in a circle or polycyclic fashion. Initially the nodules are mobile and dark-red in color. They may breakdown to form punched out ulcers or may heal leaving behind pigmentation or tissue paper-scars'. New lesions may continue to appear at the periphery-peripheral extension. They may be disposed on any part of the skin surface.

Papulosquamous/psoriasiform gummas: The lesions are similar to nodular gummata. In addition some of the lesions may show thick scales resembling psoriasis. They affect the palms and soles in addition to other parts of skin surface.

Subcutaneous gummas: They are deep seated, multiple, indurated, non-tender, discrete and firm lesions. Initially the overlying skin is normal and mobile. Later on it may adhere to these lesions, which may yield to form punched out ulcers on the skin surface, with rounded or poly-cyclic border. The older lesions heal while new lesions may continue to appear at the periphery. The walls are vertical, with the floor having dull-red granulations and yellowish-white slough-*Wash leather slough.* At the margin of the ulcer the skin is dull-red. Ulcers may be adherent to the underlying tissues namely muscles, bones, and joints. Spontaneous healing may occur leaving behind 'tissue paper scars'. They commonly affect the upper and outer one-third of the leg, below the knee , scalp, face, skin over the sternum, the sternoclavicular joints and buttocks.

Mucous membrane: The gummatous involvement of the mucous membrane presents as nodules/ ulcers and diffuse interstitial gummatous infiltration.

Gummatous nodules/ulcer: Initially a single or multiple, indurated, non-tender nodules appear over the mucous membrane, which may open to form punched out superficial or deep ulcers, arranged in polycyclic or horseshoe-shaped fashion. The margin of the ulcer is indurated, non-tender and devoid of signs of inflammation around it. In the latter the bone and cartilage underneath the ulcer may be destroyed causing a through-and-through perforation. Involvement of larynx and pharynx may lead to aphonia due to stenosis.

Diffuse interstitial gummatous infiltration: The gummatous infiltration may affect the tongue and lips. It may be asymptomatic or may present as macroglossia in the early and chronic superficial glossitis and fissured tongue in the later stages. The reporting complaint may be enlargement of the tongue. On examination the tongue may be found to be studded with irregular, white, indurated patches. The tongue may be smooth at the margins. There may be irregular fissuring of the tongue resembling scrotal skin-*scrotal tongue*. Similar type of lesions may be seen on the lips. Localized infiltration of the mucous membrane is noted in the form of grayish white, indurated, leukoplakia-like patches. They are located at the angle of mouth, on the dorsum of the tongue and the pillars of the fauces.

Table 8.3: Indications for retreatment

1. Persistence/recurrence of clinical activity of syphilis
2. Quantitative STS titers, estimated at 3-monthly intervals do not decrease at least 4-fold in 1 year.
3. Quantitative STS titer increases 4-folds, indicating relapse/reinfection.

Treat as for late syphilis

Bones: Gumma may appear mostly in the long and flat bones. The condition may be asymptomatic or associated with dull boring pain. Swellings and tenderness may be noted specially in the superficial bones, breaking open to form deep gummatous ulcers, with characteristic morphology. Radiological examination is helpful in the diagnosis. In the early lesions rarefaction and in advanced stages hypertrophic bone changes may be seen.

Viscera: Gummatous lesions may also be uncommonly found in the viscera like liver, spleen, gastrointestinal tract and testes. The involvement may be asymptomatic or the symptoms and signs may point to the involvement of these organs.

Diagnosis

It is based on the history, clinical examination and appropriate laboratory investigations. The standard serological tests are usually reactive, but non-reactive serology may not necessarily rule out the diagnosis. The specific serological tests, however, are in variably reactive. In addition radiololgical screening, and CSF examination is imperative. The therapeutic response to the specific treatment may clinch the diagnosis.

Differential Diagnosis

Gumma may have to be differentiated from nodular leprosy, acne vul-garis (conglobata), ecthyma, varicose ulcer, lupus vulgaris, sarcoidosis and erythema induratum. *Nodular leprosy* is recognized by its morphological features, complemented by the recovery of *Mycobacterium leprae* in the smear and microscopic sections of the lesions. *Acne vulgaris* (conglobata) is diagnosed by the history and the seborrhoeic distribution of the lesions. *Ecthyma* may also pose a problem. The lesions are usually painful crusted and may show excavating ulcers on removal of the crusts. The recovery of streptococci on culture may clinch the diagnosis. The diagnosis of *sarcoidosis* may be made by exclusion and predominant histiocytic granulomas, surrounded by fibrous tissue. The gummatous ulcers over the leg should be differentiated from the *varicose ulcers* and *erythema induratum*. In addition to the morphological characteristics of these ulcers, their locations on the medial side of the lower one-third of the leg and the calf respectively are the distinct pointers to their diagnosis. Likewise *lupus vulgaris* is diagnosed by its morphology (apple-jelly nodules) and histopathology. Mantoux test may be helpful.

Treatment

In the treatment of late latent syphilis and benign tertiary syphilis, the same principles are to be followed as for early syphilis. Penicillin is the drug of choice (Table 8.3).

Alternative drugs: In penicillin-sensitive patients the alternative drugs such as tetracyclines and doxycycline may be used. The CDC recommendations are outlined in Table 8.2.

Surgical intervention may be needed in cases of saddle-shaped nose, perforation of the palate and strictures of larynx and pharynx.

Follow-up

After the treatment of late latent syphilis, quantitative standard serological tests should be done at three-monthly interval for the first year, at six-monthly interval for the second year and every year for the next three years. Periodic CSF examination should be done whenever possible. It may be emphasized that the persistence of reactive standard serological tests is not an unequivocal indication for the treatment.

Table 8.4 Syphilis treatment: WHO guidelines

Early syphilis (Primary, secondary, latent syphilis of not more than 2 years duration)
Recommended regimen
Benzyl benzathine penicillin 2.4 mega unit, by intramuscular injection at a single session because of the volume involved this dose is given at two injections at separate sites
Alternative regimen
Procaine benzyl penicillin 1.2 million IU, by intramuscular injection, daily for 10 consecutive days
Alternative regimens for penicillin allergic non pregnant patients
Doxycyclline 100 mg orally twice a day for 14 days
Or
Tetracycline 500 mg orally 4 times a day for 14 days
Alternative regimens for penicillin allergic patients
Erythromycin 500 mg orally 4 times a day for 14 days
Late Latent Syphilis (Infection of more than 2 years duration without evidence of treponemal infection)
Recommended regimen
Benzyl Benzathine penicilline, 2.4 million IU, by intramuscular injection once a week for 3 consecutive weeks
Alternative regimens
Procain benzylpenicillin 1.2 million International Units, by intramuscular injection, once daily for 20 days
Alternative regimens for penicillin allergic, non pregnant patients
Doxycycline 100 mg orally twice a day for 30 days
Or
Tetracycline 500 mg orally 4 times a day for 30 days
Alternative regimens for penicillin allergic pregnant patients
Erythromycin 500 mg orally 4 times a day

It is worthwhile to consider recent recommendation of World Health Organization (WHO) guidelines to ensure its application in day-to-day practice in Table 8.4

FURTHER READING

1. Anonymous, Centre for Disease Control. Sexually transmitted diseases: treatment guidelines. MMWR 1989;38:S8.
2. Augenbraun M. Treatment of latent and tertiary syphilis. Hosp Pract (Minneap) 2000;35:89-95.
3. Augenbraun MH, Rolfs R. Treatment of syphilis, 1998: nonpregnant adults. Clin Infect Dis 1999;28: S21-8.
4. Gene M, Ledger WJ. Syphilis in pregnancy. Sex Transm Infect 2000;76:73-9.
5. Hutchinson CM, Hook EW 3rd. Syphilis in adults. Med Clin North Am 1990;74:1389-416.
6. Kumar B, Muralidhar S. Malignant syphilis: a review. AIDS Patient Care STDS 1998;12:921-5.
7. Kampmeier RH. Essentials of Syphiology (2nd edn). Oxford: Blackwell, 1946.

8. Lacey HB, Higgins SP, Graham D. An outbreak of early syphilis: Cases from North Manchester General Hospital. Sex Transm Infect. 2001;77:311-3.
9. Poulton M, Dean GI, Williams DI, Carter P, Iversen A, Fisher M. Surfing with spirochaetes: an ongoing syphilis outbreak in Brighton. Sex Transm Infect 2001;77: 319-21.
10. Palfreeman AJ, Moussa RA. Syphilis in the fens. Sex Transm Infect 2001;77:314-5.
11. Singh AE, Romanowski B. Syphilis: Review with emphasis on clinical, epidemiologic, and some biologic features. Clin Microbiol Rev 1999;12:187-209.
12. Stokes JH, Beerman H, Ingraham NR. Modern Clinical Syphiology (3rd Ed): Philadelphia: Saunders, 1945.
13. Van Voorst Vader PC. Syphilis management and treatment. Dermatol Clin 1998;16:699-711.

Chapter 9

Cardiovascular Syphilis

The involvement of the large and medium sized blood vessels and the heart is observed in late syphilis.

EPIDEMIOLOGY

About 10-15 per cent of the untreated or inadequately treated patients of syphilis may develop cardiovascular syphilis. It is more common in men than in women. It is more often noted in Negroes and manual workers. The age of onset of cardiovascular syphilis usually depends on the age at acquiring early syphilis, the time lag being 10-20 years.

PATHOGENESIS

Treponemes usually reach the cardiovascular system in the early stages of infection when there is blood-borne dissemination. Two types of reactions may be noted, gumma or diffuse interstitial inflammation. The pathogenesis of gumma is similar to that noted in the skin and the mucous membranes. Gummatous change is rarely noted in the heart.

Diffuse interstitial inflammation is noted in the large and small blood vessels. The treponemes reach the aortic wall through the vasa vasorum during the early stages of infection and remain dormant for a varying period. Slowly an inflammatory reaction consisting of lymphocytes and plasma cells is noted around the vasa vasorum. Endarteritic changes result in necrosis and subsequent fibrosis of the part of the media supplied by those vessels. The intimal layer in proximity to these patches may show thickening. In the later stages the adventitia also becomes fibrotic leading to loss of elasticity of the aortic wall. The dilatation of the aortic wall is noted because of the continuous high pressure and loss of elasticity. If the dilatation is in the proximal part of aorta, the aortic ring is involved with separation of the cusps and subsequent aortic regurgitation. The valves also may become fibrotic. Both the coronary ostia may be involved, and get narrowed.

CLINICAL FEATURES

The cardiovascular syphilis may manifest as aortitis, aortic aneurysm, aortic insufficiency (regurgitation) and coronary insufficiency. Occasionally, myocarditis and affliction of the medium blood vessels, may be seen.

Aortitis

It is usually asymptomatic, but in some it may be accompanied by symptoms. The patient may present with burning or substernal pain, paroxysmal or exertional dyspnea. Examination of the chest may reveal episternal pulsations, increasing dullness over the manubrium sterni, accen-tuation of second aortic sound and systolic murmur in aortic area. The fluoroscopic evidence of aortic dilatation may be contributory to its diagnosis.

Aortic Aneurysm

The dilatation of the aorta is called aortic aneurysm. It may be fusiform or saccular. Syphilis usually affects the ascending aorta, the arch of aorta and parts of thoracic aorta. Other parts of the aorta may also be involved. The aneurysm may be asymptomatic or may present the clinical features, according to the involvement of different part of the aorta. Spontaneous rupture of aneurysm of the aorta may cause sudden death.

Aneurysm of Ascending Aorta (Aneurysm of Signs)

The patient presents with dull boring retrosternal pain and pulsations in the aortic area. Sometimes pressure symptoms may be noted. Examination may show low blood pressure on the right arm as compared to the left. A pulsating swelling may be seen in and around the manubrium sterni. A systolic thrill with a systolic murmur in the aortic area, radiating to the cervical arteries, is classic. It is at times associated with aortic regurgitation *(vide infra).*

Aneurysm of the Arch of Aorta (Aneurysm of Symptoms)

Aneurysm of arch of aorta manifests as a pulsating swelling in the suprasternal area (Figs 9.1 and 9.2) or in addition it may have features pointing to the compression of the surrounding structures such astrachea. The patient may present with brassy cough, dyspnea and recurrent pulmonary infections. The tracheal tug may be elicited in case of pressure on the left bronchus. Recurrent laryngeal nerve. The patient may report with hoarseness of voice due to paralysis of the left vocal cord.

- *Esophagus:* It may cause dysphagia.
- *Superior vena cava:* It may lead to edema of the face and engorgement of the veins on the chest, neck and arms. It may also be associated with cyanosis.
- *Cervical sympathetic chain* The involvement of the cervical sympathetic chain on the left side may manifest as *'Horner's syndrome'*, characterized by enophthalmos, miosis, and impairment or loss of sweating on the left side of the face.
- *Vertebrae:* The aneurysm may cause erosion of the vertebrae, presenting as dull, boring retrosternal pain.
- *Innominate artery:* The affliction of this artery may cause dizziness, variation in systolic pressure, and asynchrony of the radial pulse.

Aneurysm of Descending Aorta (Asymptomatic Aneurysm)

It is of rare occurrence and is usually asymptomatic. Occasional dull aching or boring pain may be the only presenting complaint.

Diagnosis: It is based on the history, the cardinal clinical features, the fluoroscopy and radiograms comprising X-ray chest, barium-swallow and aortogram. Serological diagnosis of syphilis is, however, imperative. Aortic aneurysm due to atherosclerosis needs to be considered in differential diagnosis.

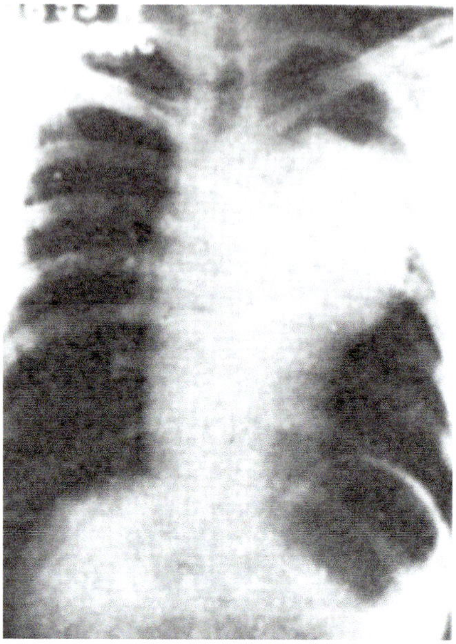

Fig. 9.1: Cardiovascular syphilis. Aneurysm of the arch of aorta, anteroposterior view

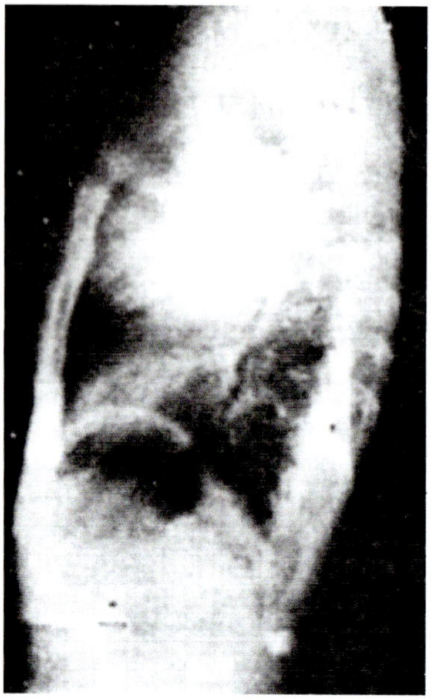

Fig. 9.2: Cardiovascular syphilis. Aneurysm of the arch of aorta, lateral view

Aortic Insufficiency

It may be asymptomatic with exertional or paroxysmal nocturnal dyspnea, angina pectoris, palpitation, vertigo and syncopal attack. Examination of the heart on palpation may show the shifting of the apex beat downwards and to the left with a hyperdynamic forceful thrust. The diastolic murmur on auscultation of the aortic area is the cardinal sign. It is an early, high pitched, decrescendo diastolic murmur, soft, and blowing with or after the second sound or masking the sound completely. It is audible all over the precordium, but is best heard in the aortic area or in the left third or fourth parasternal space with the patient leaning forward. The simultaneous systolic and diastolic murmurs- *to and fro or sea-saw murmurs,* due to aneurysm of the aorta and aortic regurgitation may also be noted.

In addition, the condition is recognised by the presence of cardinal signs in the peripheral blood vessels. They are characterized by *water hammer or collapsing* (Corrigan) pulse, marked pulsations in the neck vessels (dancing carotids, Corrigan's sign), low diastolic and wide pulse pressure, the difference of blood pressures noted between the femoral and brachial arteries being more than 20 mm of Hg (Hill's sign), capillary pulsations, the pistol-shot sounds over the femoral arteries (Traube's sign) and the diastolic murmur over the femoral artery heard on pressing the artery about 2 cm below the stethoscope (Duroziez's sign).

Diagnosis It is based on the history and the cardinal clinical features. The radiogram may show a boot-shaped heart due to enlargement of the left ventricle. Similarly, electrocardiogram may reveal left ventricular hypertrophy with diastolic overload pattern. The syphilitic aortic regurgitation may have to be differentiated from atherosclerotic, congenital, and Marfan's syndrome.

Coronary Insufficiency

The affection of the mouths of the coronary arteries in syphilitic aortic insufficiency may cause symptoms of angina pectoris. Pain characterizes angina pectoris. It is usually substernal or apical, radiated to the left arm, the neck and the jaw. Initially pain may be of constricting or choking type, appearing on exertion and disappearing on rest. However, the attack of pain may occur even on rest as the condition progresses. The attack of pain usually lasts for a short period to reappear again. Occasionally it may be massive and cause myocardial infarction, especially when associated with atheroma. Emotional upset, such as fear and anger may precipitate the disease.

It may be associated with an inability to breathe, choking sensation, belching or passage of flatus, dizziness and fainting. Clinical examination during the attack may not reveal any signs or pallor, sweating and fall of blood pressure, often associated with tachycardia, may be seen. Pressure on the carotid sinus may produce slowing of pulse and cessation of pain.

Diagnosis: It is made by the classical presenting features. Electrocardiogram may contribute towards the diagnosis. The characteristic changes in the electrocardiogram may be depression of the ST segment and inversion of the T-wave. These changes may at times be noted when the electrocardiogram is taken after exertion only (Fig. 9.3). Glyceryl trinitrate (0.5 mg) tablet sublingually may relieve angina pectoris. Hence, it is used as a therapeutic test. Serological diagnosis of syphilis is, however, imperative.

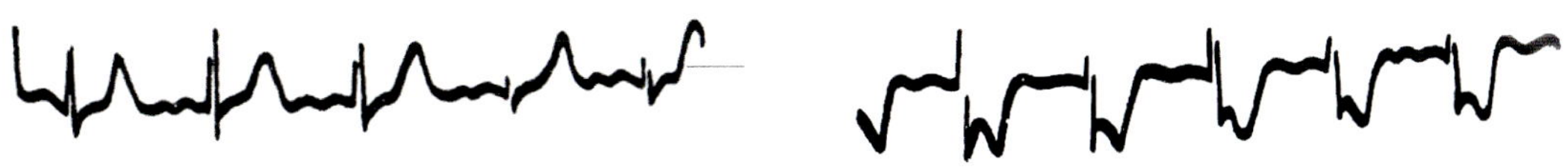

Figs. 9.3A and B: Electrocardiogram showing changes at rest (A) and after exertion (B), wherein depression of the ST segment and inversion of the T-wave are evident

Myocarditis

It is a rare situation. Occasionally, gummatous myocarditis may be encountered.

The involvement of the medium sized blood vessels occasionally may also be seen. Accordingly, symptoms and signs of affected organ are noted.

Treatment

It consists of giving penicillin in the recommended dosage in a schedule, similar to that of late syphilis. It may be emphasized that with this treatment only further damage to the organ can be arrested, but the damage already present may not be reversible. Moreover, at times the treatment may further complicate the condition, due to therapeutic response, therapeutic *paradox.*

General line of treatment will, however, depend on the organ involved and the extent of the damage.

FURTHER READING

1. Kuniyoshi Y, Koja K, Miyagi K, Shimoji M, Kudaka M, Uezu T, et al. A ruptured syphilitic descending thoracic aortic aneurysm. The characteristic findings on computed tomography for the etiological diagnosis of aneurysm. Ann Thorac Cardiovasc Surg 1998;4:99-102.
2. Stokes JH, Beerman H, Ingraham NR. Modern Clinical Syphiology (3rd edn). Philadelphia: Saunders, 1945.

Chapter 10

Neurosyphilis

INTRODUCTION

Syphilis, in the early as well as late stages, may affect the nervous system with or without manifesting clinical features.

EPIDEMIOLOGY

About 12.5 percent of the untreated or inadequately treated patients of early and late syphilis may develop neurosyphilis. The age of onset of late neurosyphilis usually depends upon the age at acquiring early syphilis, its duration being 8-10 years. It is more common in men than in women. It occurs at a greater frequency amongst white as compared to black races.

PATHOGENESIS

Treponema pallidum may invade the nervous system in early syphilis, evidence of which may only be seen in cerebrospinal fluid (CSF)—asymptomatic neurosyphilis. The organisms may lie dormant for a considerable time after which the classical inflammatory reaction may set in, affecting the various tissues such as the meninges, the blood vessels and the parenchyma of the brain and the spinal cord. The pathological changes in the meninges are characterized by perivascular infiltrate consisting largely of lymphocytes and plasma cells usually affecting the pia and the arachnoid layers. Later, fibrotic changes may be seen. Side by side subependymal gliosis may also be seen. These changes usually affect the meninges of the vertex, base of the brain, cervical and dorsolumbar region, giving rise to different manifestations.

The medium sized blood vessels of the brain and the spinal cord may also be affected. The microscopic pathology is akin to syphilitic aortitis. The narrowing of the lumen because of the thickening of the vessel wall may lead to thrombosis, causing infarction of the affected part of the parenchyma. Middle, anterior and posterior cerebral arteries, posterior-inferior cerebellar, basilar and spinal arteries are also affected.

Changes in the parenchyma of the brain may also be seen. They are characterized by degenerative changes involving the ganglion cells, the axon cylinders and the myelin sheath. There may be hypertrophy of the glial tissue along with proliferation of the histiocytes and infiltration by the lymphocytes and the plasma cells in the cortex. The iron laden histiocytes are pathognomonic of involvement of the parenchyma. *Treponema pallidum* may also be demonstrated by the special staining. The involvement of the parenchyma is usually associated with inflammation of the meninges. The meninges may be thickened with the pia mater firmly adherent to the cortex, with a dilated subarachnoid space. The cerebral convolutions are firm and flattened, because of atrophy and fibrosis. The ventricular system may be dilated with ependymal gliosis.

The spinal cord may be affected in a similar fashion as the brain. However, the brunt of the disease is borne by the posterior columns of the spinal cord showing atrophy and infiltration by the lymphocytes and plasma cells.

Optic nerve may also be affected resulting in primary optic atrophy.

CLASSIFICATION

Treponema pallidum may affect the brain and/or the spinal cord resulting in various lesions, manifesting in different ways as shown in Table 10.1.

Table 10.1: Classification

Asymptomatic	No signs/symptoms	CSF changes only
Meningeal	Cerebral	Acute, subacute or chronic meningitis affecting the vertex or the base of the brain
	Spinal	Hypertrophic cervical pachymeningitis, doroslumbar meningitis and amyotrophic lateral sclerosis
Vascular	Cerebral	Syphilitic vascular thrombosis leading to various syndromes depending upon arteries involved.
	Spinal	Syphilitic vascular thrombosis leading to paraplegia below the level of involvement.
	Cerebral	General paralysis of insane.
Parenchymatous		Primary optic atrophy.
	Spinal	Tabes dorsalis.
Gumma	Cerebral	Symptoms and signs of space occupying lesion.
	Spinal	Symptoms and signs of space occupying lesion.

ASYMPTOMATIC NEUROSYPHILIS

Apparently there are no clinical symptoms and signs suggestive of the involvement of the nervous system in a syphilitic patient. The diagnosis of this condition is made by the changes in cerebrospinal fluid (CSF) which are, an increase in lymphocytes—more than five lymphocytes per mm^3, increase in total proteins (IgG and IgM) beyond 40 mg percent, and reactive qualitative/quantitative serological tests for syphilis.

GENERAL PARALYSIS OF INSANE

In general paralysis of insane (GPI), there is an insidious involvement of the parenchyma of the brain by *Treponema pallidum*. The presenting feature being a progressive deterioration of all the mental faculties, characterized by dementia around which a variety of accessory psychiatric and neurologic manifestations are formed.

Clinical Features

The onset of the disease is usually insidious. The disease may be divided into various stages, such as incipient stage, period of full development and period of decline. At times, it may be hard to differentiate one stage from another, for the clinical features of one may overlap the other.

Incipient Stage

It may present in the form of changes in personality and progressive deterioration of mental faculties. Initially, there may be impairment or loss of memory and a complete disorientation of time, place and person. The patient may become apathetic and dull. Occasionally, the onset of the disease may be sudden, characterized by convulsive seizures, monoplegias, hemiplegias, aphasia or short period of mental confusion. These changes may be transient. They may be followed by changes in the psychiatric behavior.

Period of Full Development

It may be present as variegated psychosis. It may either be simple dementia marked by memory defects, impairment or loss of judgement and instability of mood. It may present as grandiose type characterized by euphoria and expressions of delusions of grandeur—classical type, though uncommon manifestations like manic-depressive psychosis, paranoid and schizophrenia may also be observed.

Period of decline The patient may pass onto this stage with the preceding symptoms becoming conspicuous. The epileptiform or apoplectic seizures may follow, resulting in further deterioration of the condition. The patient may develop incontinence of urine and may become bed-ridden. The examination of the patient may reveal the following:

Mental status The consecutive record of the mental status of the patient may show deterioration.

Speech It may manifest as dysarthria, hesitancy and slurring.

Ocular changes The pupillary changes consist of irregularity of outline, inequality of size and impairment or loss of light reflex. There may be associated oculomotor palsy and optic atrophy. *Argyll-Robertson pupil* may be classical.

Handwriting It may show misspelt words and omissions, misplacements and repetitions of letters and syllables. There may be agraphia in the late stages. The record of handwriting may be useful in the progress of the condition (Fig. 10.1).

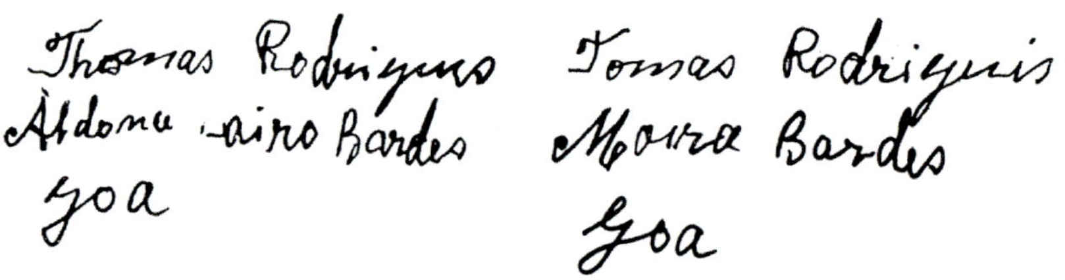

Fig. 10.1: Handwriting of GPI

Face The face may be expressionless. There may be flattening and smoothening out of nasolabial folds. Tremors of the lips and tongue may be present. In the terminal stages the disease may progress to generalized spasticity and a decerebrate attitude.

Reflexes The deep reflexes like the ankle-and knee jerks are exaggerated, while superficial reflexes such as abdominal may be lost and plantars are extensors.

Diagnosis

The diagnosis is based on the history, the presenting clinical features, the CSF finding and the serological tests for syphilis. Cerebrospinal fluid examination usually shows increased cell count, moderate increase in lymphocytes, increase in proteins and first zone type of colloidal gold curve (paretic curve). The standard and the specific serological tests done on CSF are reactive. The blood serology is also imperative in its diagnosis (Table 10.2).

Table 10.2: Cerebrospinal fluid in neurosyphilis

Classification	*Cells*	*Proteins*	*CSF and STS*	*Colloidal gold curve*	*STS blood*
Normal	0-5 lymphocytes	30-40 mg	Non-reactive	Normal	Non-reactive
Asymptomatic	Increased	Increased	Reactive/ non-reactive	First zone/normal	Reactive/ non-reactive
Meningeal	Increased/50%	Increased/normal	Reactive 65%	Midzone	Reactive 80%
Vascular	Increased/normal	Increased/normal	Reactive/ non-reactive	Normal	Reactive
Parenchymatous GPI	Increased	Increased	Reactive	First zone Paretic curve	Reactive 95%
Tabes dorsalis	Increased/normal	Increased/normal	Reactive/ non-reactive	First zone/midzone	Reactive/ non-reactive
Gumma	Increased/normal	Increased/normal	Reactive/ non-reactive	Normal	Reactive

It may have to be distinguished from other psychotic and psychoneurotic conditions due to *atherosclerosis, senility, alcoholism, drugs, toxemia,* etc.

TABES DORSALIS

It is a progressive degeneration of the posterior columns of the spinal cord and atrophy of the dorsal roots, with presenting clinical features pointing to their involvement.

Clinical Features

It may present in various clinical ways, but subjective sensory disturbances characterized by lightening pains, fixed pains, girdle pains and the pains of tabetic crises are classical. Tabetic crises are paroxysmal painful disorders of functions of various viscera—the gastric crises being the most common. It is characterized by attacks of epigastric pain associated with severe vomiting, lasting for a few hours to several days. Laryngeal, rectal and vesicles crises have also been described. The patient may also complain of a feeling of walking on cotton wool. Side-by-side difficulty in micturition and an overflow incontinence of urine, may be present. Incontinence may sometimes be an early symptom. In addition ataxia is a prominent presenting complaint. The examination may reveal the following signs.

Sensations Superficial sensations are lost on the butterfly area of the face, inner sides of the arms, saddle-shaped area around the anus and lateral aspects or stocking areas of the lower limbs. Deep sensations such as deep pains, vibration and joint sense are usually lost in the lower limbs.

Reflexes An asymmetrical diminution of deep reflexes is the earliest sign. However, the early loss of the ankle jerks is a consistent feature. The abdominal reflexes are lost in the late stages due to atonia of the muscles, but the plantars are always flexors.

Ataxia Ataxic gait is characteristic, that is the patient walks on a wide base, eyes fixed to the ground, legs lifted unduly in the air and brought down with a stamp (stamping gait). *Romberg's sign* is usually positive—inability to stand upright with the feet together and the eyes closed.

Trophic changes They may be present as perforating ulcers located usually at the base of the great toe or as Charcot's joints. *Charcot's joint* is characterized by effusion, hypermobility and various types of deformities due to destructive changes. Usually a single joint is affected, the knee joint being the most common. The radiogram reveals erosion, rarefaction, destruction of joint surfaces and new bone formation. At times fracture dislocation may also be seen.

Ocular changes The pupils are irregular and unequal in size. Their reaction to light is sluggish. *Argyll-Robertson pupil* when found is classical. It is characterized by small, irregular, unequal pupils which do not react to light, but contract on accommodation.

Primary optic atrophy It is classical clinical manifestation of tabes dorsalis observed in some patients. It is initially evident in the form of diminution of vision with progressive narrowing of the visual fields. It may lead to complete blindness.

Ophthalmoscopy may reveal a greyish-white atrophic cup-shaped optic disk. The lamina cribrosa may show stippling.

Bladder It becomes large and atonic. Catheterization usually reveals a few ounces of residual urine.

Diagnosis

It is made by the triad of symptoms of lightening pains, dysuria and ataxia, complemented by the triad of signs, *Argyll-Robertson pupil,* absent tendon reflexes and positive *Romberg's sign.* It is invariably confirmed by the cerebrospinal fluid examination, which indicates lymphocytosis, increase in IgG and IgM and reactive standard as well as specific serological tests for syphilis (Table 10.2). In burnt out cases of tabes dorsalis, the CSF findings may not show any abnormalities.

The condition needs differentiation from other neurological conditions such as *subacute combined degeneration, disseminated sclerosis, syringomyelia, Friedreich's ataxia* and *chronic polyneuritis.*

TABOPARESIS

The parenchymatous involvement of the brain and the spinal cord may simultaneously be seen in the same patient with signs and symptoms of GPI and tabes dorsalis *(vide supra).*

MENINGEAL SYPHILIS

The meninges may be affected in early as well as late syphilis. The clinical manifestations may either be acute, subacute or chronic.

Acute meningitis It is characterized by symptoms of increased intracranial pressure like headache, nausea and vomiting. The *Kernig's sign* suggestive of meningeal irritation, may be positive. Cranial nerve palsies may also be seen.

Subacute and chronic meningitis It is due to the involvement of meninges of the base of the brain. It may result in uni- or bilateral cranial nerve palsies mainly affecting the third, sixth, seventh and eighth nerves. The focal signs, suggestive of involvement of these nerves, may be positive. In addition there may be signs and symptoms of raised intracranial tension due to obstruction. *Argyll-Robertson pupil* may also be noted.

Spinal cord meninges may rarely be affected and may result in different syndromes.

Cervical hypertrophic pachymeningitis It is characterized by pain in the neck radiating down the upper limbs and between the shoulders. Further, lower motor neurone type of involvement of the shoulder girdle muscles is noted.

Erb's spastic paraplegia It is characterized by upper motor neurone type of involvement of the extensor muscles of the legs, with an early involvement of the bladder causing frequency of micturition.

Amyotrophic lateral sclerosis A combination of certain features of the preceding conditions are noted in this syndrome.

Diagnosis

In addition to the clinical features, the diagnosis is made by CSF examination (Table 10.2).

VASCULAR SYPHILIS

The blood vessels of the brain may be affected in syphilis. Depending upon the affected vessels, various clinical syndromes may result. Focalization of the lesion is determined by the site and the extent of infarction of the brain. Usually the onset is sudden, associated with giddiness and motor paralysis such as aphasia, monoplegia and hemiplegia. Similar type of changes may be noticed in the spinal cord, giving rise to paraplegia due to involvement of the spinal cord at different sites.

GUMMA

They mainly affect meninges resulting in focal cerebral meningeal neurosyphilis with signs of a space occupying lesion and abnormality in the cerebrospinal fluid.

Treatment

Penicillin is the mainstay in the treatment of neurosyphilis. It is, however, imperative to emphasize that penicillin must be given in adequate dosage at the earliest opportunity as soon as the diagnosis is made. Moreover, the specific treatment is useful only in arresting the progress of syphilis, but the damage already done may not be reversible.

At times, with the specific line of treatment, instead of normal anticipated improve-ment or cure, worsening of the condition is noted due to thera-peutic response-*therapeutic paradox.*

The CDC recommendation for treatment are detailed in Table 10.3.

Table 10.3: Neurosyphilis treatment: CDC recommendcition

Aqueous crystalline penicillin G, 12-24 million units, IV daily (2-4 million units IV, every four hours) for 10 to 14 days
Or
Procaine penicillin G, 2.4 million units IM daily for 10 to 14 days
With
500 mg of probenecid, four times a day
Followed by
2.4 million units of Benzathine penicillin G, IM, every week for 3 weeks (Total of 7.2 million units)

Follow-up

It is carried out in the same fashion as for late syphilis. Additionally, CSF examination may be done following the specific treatment, at an interval of six months in order to judge the progress of the condition. The success of the treatment is indicated by the reversal and maintenance of the cell count to normal in the follow-up examination. Retreatment is indicated if there is a persistently high cell count in the CSF, increase in the CSF proteins and a rising serological titer. Also when there is a persistent increase in cell count—lymphocytes more than 5 per mm3 alone—suggest activity of neurosyphilis and is an indication for retreatment *(Dattner-Thomas concept)* (Table 10.4). Reactive serology may, however, continue for a longer period, but is never an indication for retreatment.

Recent World Health Organization (WHO) guidelines for the treatment are included to facilitate option Table 10.5

The central nervous system may be involved during any stage of syphilis. Clinical evidence of neurological involvement in the form of (auditory symptoms or cranial nerve palsies), warrants examination of the CNS. However, examination of CNS is desirable in all those patients with syphilis of more than 2 years duration or of uncertain duration, in order to evaluate for the possible presence

Table 10.4: Assessment of activity of neurosyphilis *(Dattner-Thomas concept with modifications)*

1. Syphilitic infection may be very active within the central nervous system and yet be asymptomatic; Signs and symptoms are not reliable indicators of the activity
2. A reactive spinal fluid non-treponemal test alone is not a proof of active neurosyphilis; Increased cell counts and total protein determinations are more reliable indicators of activity
3. In an arrested case of neurosyphilis, cell counts should become normal within 3 to 4 months after treatment, while quantitative non-treponemal tests and protein values show a gradual and steady trend to normal
4. Following specific therapy with penicillin for active neurosyphilis, the spinal fluid may show a trend towards normal, only to relapse later; Relapses, however, rarely occur more than 1 year following therapy; If the cell count is not normal and no improvement occurs in total protein and quantitative non-treponemal tests 6 months after treatment, further treatment is imperative, regardless of the clinical status of the patient
5. A reactive CSF-IgM-TPHA test indicates active infection
6. A CSF-TPHA index above 100 is suggestive of active neurosyphilis, provided the albumin quotient does not exceed 20
7. A nonreactive CSF-FTA-ABS and/or CSF-TPHA usually excludes neurosyphilis

* A measure of the permeability of blood-brain barrier

Table 10.5: Neurosyphilis treatment: WHO guidelines

Recommended regimen

Aqueous benzyl penicillin 1.2 -2.4 million units by intravenous injection administered daily in a dose of 2-4 million units every 4 hours for 14 days

Alternative regimen

Procaine benzyle penicillin 1.2 million IU, daily by intramuscular injection , once daily and probenecid 500 mg orally 4 times daily, both for 14 days.
This regimen should be used for only those patients whose outpatient compliance can be assured.
Some authorities recommend adding benzathine benzyl penicilline 2.4 million IU by intramuscular injection in 3 consecutive doses once weekly after completing this regimen, but there are no data to support this approach. Benzathine benzyl penicillin 2.4 million units does not give adequate therapeutic levels in the CSF.

Alternative regimens for penicillin allergic, non pregnant patients

Doxycycline 200 mg orally twice a day for 30 days
Or Erythromycin 500 mg, 4 times a day for 30 days.

Note: The above alternatives to penicillin have not been evaluated in systemic studies. Although their efficacy is still not known, third generation cephalosporins may be useful in the treatment of neurosyphilis

of asymptomatic neurosyphilis. Some experts recommend consulting a neurologist while caring for a patient of neurosyphilis. Careful follow-up is essential.

FURTHER READING

1. Anonymous: Centre for disease control: Sexually transmitted diseases: treatment guidelines MMWR 1989;38:S8.
2. Dattner B, Thomas EW. The management of neurosphilis. Heinemann: London, 1944.
3. Hooshmand H, Escobar MR, Kopl SW. Neurosyphilis. A study of 241 patients. JAMA 1972;219:726-9.
4. Hotson JR. Modern neurosyphilis: a partially treated chronic meningitis. West J Med 1981;135:191-200.
5. Lukehart SA, Hook EW 3rd, Baker-Zander SA, Collier AC, Critchlow CW, Handsfield HH. Invasion of the central nervous system by *Treponema pallidum*. Implications for diagnosis and treatment. Ann Int Med 1988;109:855-62.
6. Merritt HH, Moore M. Acute syphilitic meningitis. Medicine 1935;14:119-83.
7. Mills CH. Routine examination of the cerebrospinal fluid in syphilis: its value in regard to more accurate knowledge, prognosis, and treatment. Br Med J 1927;2:527-31.

Chapter 11

Congenital Syphilis

INTRODUCTION

Congenital syphilis is an infection of the fetus *in utero,* transmitted by the syphilitic mother, through the placenta or from the uterine wall resulting in miscarriage, stillbirth or a live syphilitic child.

EPIDEMIOLOGY

It is hard to get the precise incidence of congenital syphilis from different countries of the world. Nevertheless, it seems that the occurrence of the disease is considerably on the decline, in India as well as in other developed and underdeveloped countries. This may possibly be attributed to the meticulous antenatal check-up, improved diagnostic procedures, and institution of prompt and necessary therapeutic measures in pregnant mothers in most countries. The disease occurs both in males and females, during infancy and childhood.

PATHOGENESIS

The infection is transmitted through the placental circulation of the syphilitic mother *in utero* to the fetus. This usually occurs between the fourth and sixth month of pregnancy through the degenerating Langhans' layer of the placenta. The organisms disseminate and multiply in the various organs of the fetus causing an inflammatory reaction. The fate of the fetus depends upon the severity of the infection, pathological damage, and stage of infection in the mother. Hence, it may result in miscarriage, stillbirth or a child is born with congenital syphilis. It is interesting to emphasize that the performance of the pregnant mother improves with each subsequent pregnancy so that a normal child may ultimately be delivered—**Kassowitz's law**. Furthermore, it is significant to remember that a congenital syphilitic infant cannot infect its own mother, although transmission of infection to another person (wet nurse) may be possible—**Colles' law**. The treponemes in the infant continue to multiply in the different organs including the skin and the mucous membrane, rapidly setting in a cellular inflammatory reaction similar to that of secondary stage of acquired syphilis. It is characterized by infiltration of lymphocytes and plasma cells in the perivascular lymphatics. The tissue reaction results in proliferation and hypertrophy of the endothelium of the capillaries resulting in endarteritis obliterans. These changes manifest in the form of polymorphic lesions over the skin characterized by induration and necrosis.

The late manifestations of the disease are characterized by gummas affecting various organs. It represents a hypersensitivity reaction to the organisms which is evident by their absence and its successful response to the antisyphilitic treatment. Pathology of these lesions is marked by central caseation necrosis surrounded by infiltration of lymphocytes and plasma cells. The infiltrate is conspicuous around the blood vessels in the form of perivascular cuffing. Occasionally, epithelioid and giant cells are seen at the periphery with surrounding extensive fibrosis.

Similarly, the pathological changes may appear in any of the organs such as—lymph node, liver, spleen, eyes, bones, joints in addition to the central nervous system. Occasionally, the cardiovascular system may also be affected.

CLASSIFICATION

The clinical course of congenital syphilis can arbitrarily be divided into early congenital syphilis, lasting for a period of two years and late congenital syphilis occurring after an interval of two years. The early/late manifestations of congenital syphilis may leave behind stigmata.

Early Congenital Syphilis

Clinical Features

The primary stage is conspicuous by its absence. The child may either be born with manifestations of the disease or apparently normal, to manifest the disease couple of weeks later. It may be full term or premature. It is usually underweight, emaciated, marasmic and of cafe-au-lait tinge with wrinkled skin resembling that of an old man. The skin is dry and scaly. The abdomen is protuberant.

The eruptions in the child may be confined to the skin and/or mucous membranes (Table 11.1).

Skin: The vesiculobullous eruptions of the skin and mucous membranes are the hallmark of the disease at birth. The bullae are multiple, discrete, tense, 2-3 cm in size present over an apparently normal skin. They may contain serous or seropurulent fluid. They may burst leaving behind erythematous, elevated and indurated erosions. They are mainly located on the palms and soles (Fig. 11.1) and also on the face especially around the oral cavity, the trunk, the buttocks and the genitalia. They are bilateral and symmetrical.

A few weeks later a polymorphic rash predominantly of papulosquamous eruptions (Fig. 11.2) resembling syphilids of secondary stage of acquired syphilis may appear. These eruptions may be distributed on the face particularly around the mouth, buttocks, palms and soles.

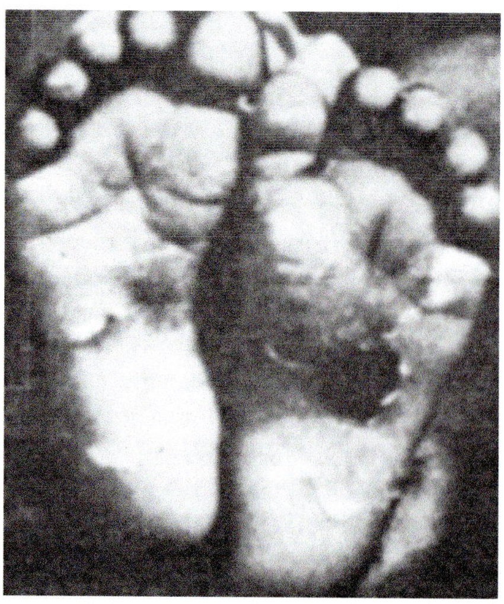

Fig. 11.1: Congenital syphilis. Vesiculobullous eruptions on the sole of the foot with indurated erosions

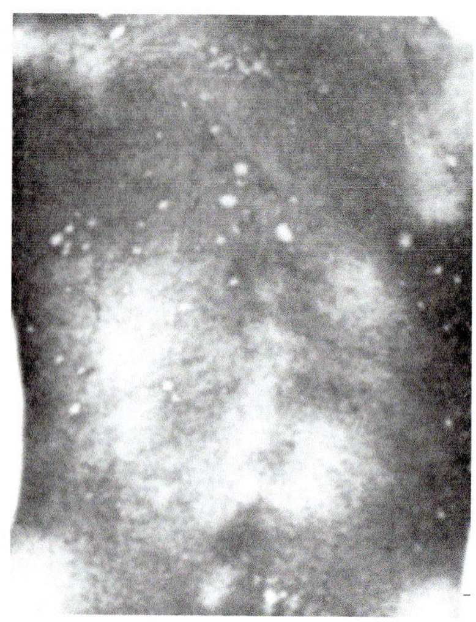

Fig. 11.2: Congenital syphilis. Papulosquamous eruption

Table 11.1: Early congenital syphilis

1. Serous/seropurulent bullous eruptions over the palms and soles, rich in *T. pallidum*, bilateral and symmetrical
2. Syphilids, like eruption namely papular, papulosquamous and condylomata lata
3. Linear radiating fissures at the angle of the mouth, perianal, and about the nares
4. Old man's look and *cafe-au-lait* tinge of the skin may be striking
5. Patchy irregular loss of hair, at the sides and back of the scalp, 'moth-eaten alopecia'
6. Syphilitic onychia
7. 'Syphilitic snuffles' is cardinal; Mucosae of the oral cavity, throat, and genitals may also be affected
8. Generalized lymphadenopathy, marked by discrete, firm, rubbery, mobile lymph nodes
9. Hepatosplenomegaly, white-pneumonia, orchitis, albuminuria, choroidoretinitis and osteochondritis of long bones (pseudoparalysis)

Condylomata lata Characterized by broad-based, hypertrophic, flat-topped, greyish-white, moist papules distributed over the angle of the mouth, the nostrils, the vulva and around the anus may be seen. They may get infected to form radiating scars—*syphilitic rhagades* (Fig. 11.3) around the oral cavity and the anus. *Follicular syphilids* resulting in patchy alopecia may also appear on the scalp. The nailbeds and folds may be affected causing *syphilitic onychia.*

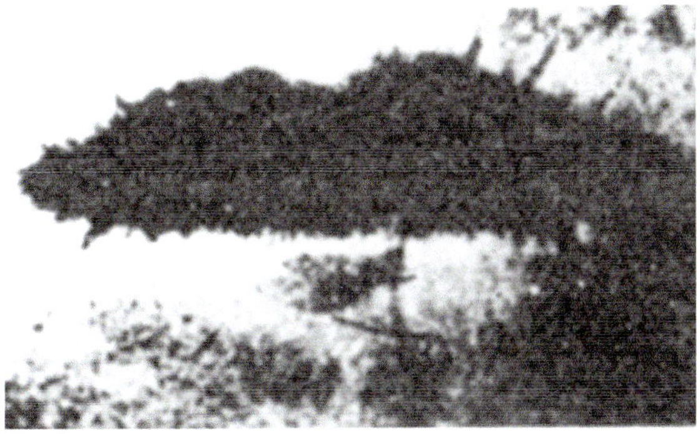

Fig. 11.3: Congenital syphilis. Syphilitic rhagades (*Courtesy:* Dr CP Hornstein and Dr RJ Gortin, The CV Mosby Co, USA)

Mucous membrane The mucous membrane lesions are quite typical. They are smooth, greyish-white *mucous patches* involving the palate, the tongue, the pharynx and the larynx. They may get eroded to form erosions or classical 'snail-track' *ulcers.* Similar lesions may also be seen in the nostrils affecting mucoperiosteum of the nasal septum, causing nasal discharge and obstruction responsible for syphilitic 'snuffles'. Later it may produce the *saddle-shaped* nose in consequence to impaired or improper growth of the nasal bone. The affection of the mucous membrane of the larynx may cause obstruction and give rise to a peculiar cry in the newborn—*syphilitic aphonia.*

Bones Osteochondritis is the earliest characteristic involvement of the bones. It affects the growing ends of long bones, namely the tibia, the radius and the ulna. Clinically,it may be asymptomatic or the child may not move the legs because of pain-syphilitic *pseudoparalysis.* The radiological examination is helpful in its diagnosis. It is marked by *saw-teeth* appearance of epiphyses and a thin radiopaque line on the surface of the cortex of the bone (Fig. 11.4). Occasionally, even the separation of the epiphyses or its fracture may be seen. Later in the course of the disease the child may present with *dactylitis* affecting the phalanges with the formation of fusiform swellings due to

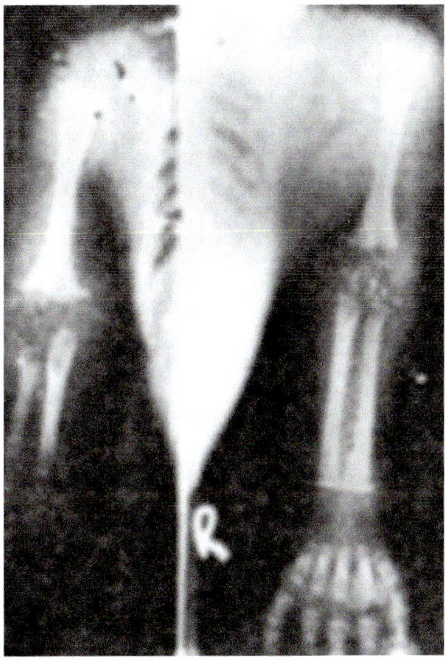

Fig. 11.4: Congenital syphilis. Bone changes (*Courtesy:* Dr PN Rangiah)

osteoperiostitis. Rarefaction and new bone formation may also occur in other long bones. The continuation of periostitis may lead to new bone formation in successive layers on the surface of the cortex, giving an *onion-peel appearance* radiologically.

Lymph nodes Generalized lymphadenopathy may be a feature. The clinical features of these glands are typical. They are multiple, nontender, discrete, firm and mobile.

Viscera The other organs like liver, spleen, kidneys and lungs may also get involved. There may be mild-to-severe hepatosplenomegaly. It may be associated with signs of jaundice and hypoproteinemia. The abdomen may be protuberant because of ascites. The involvement of the kidneys may be evident by the presence of albumin and casts in the urine due to infiltration of the glomeruli. There is no clinical evidence of lung involvement, but diffuse infiltration of the lung parenchyma-white pneumonia may be seen at autopsy.

Central nervous system The involvement of the central nervous system is rare and is similar to that in acquired secondary syphilis. When it occurs it is usually asymptomatic. Occasionally, symptomatic neurosyphilis is also encountered. In asymptomatic neurosyphilis certain cerebrospinal fluid (CSF) abnormalities are recorded without any apparent clinical features, while in symptomatic neurosyphilis symptoms and signs suggestive of meningeal involvement showing increased intracranial tension are seen in addition to the CSF findings. Occasionally, hydrocephalus may be noted. The CSF examination in these patients shows increase in globulin-IgG and IgM, lymphocytes and a reactive serology (see Table 10.2).

Eyes They are rarely affected. Choroidoretinitis being one of them, which may leave behind stigma—*pepper* and *salt* fundus.

Table 11.2: Late congenital syphilis

1. 'Gumma' is cardinal
2. Interstitial keratitis, marked by pain and photophobia may affect both eyes, either simultaneously or successively; corneal scarring (ghost-vessels) may be sequelae
3. Bilateral progressive perceptive deafness may have an onset in the middle-age
4. Neurological manifestations characterized by asymptomatic meningeal/vascular/parenchymatous/neurosyphilis
5. Skeletal involvement; characterized by gummatous osteoperiostitis (5-20 years); sabre tibia, parrots nodes, saddle nose, perforated nasal septum, thickening of inner end of clavicle (Higoumenakis'sign)
6. Clutton's joints (painless, insidious, swelling of joints especially knee)
7. Paroxysmal cold hemoglobinuria cardiovascular syphilis and visceral gummata may be other uncommon manifestations

Diagnosis

It is based on the history, the clinical manifestations and on the demonstration of *T. pallidum* under the dark ground microscope by the regular wet preparation or by the direct fluorescent technique. The material for the test is obtained from vesiculobullous eruptions, erosions, ulcers, condylomata lata lesions and the lymph glands. The standard and the specific serological tests when positive in the cord blood may either be because of antibodies acquired from the mother or the antibodies produced by the infected infant. The rising titre of the standard quantitative tests indicates infection in the infant, while the falling titre indicates the presence of maternal antibodies. Furthermore, the diagnosis of congenital syphilis is clinched by the demonstration of reactive FTA-ABS (IgM) test. The IgM antibodies when present belong only to the infant, for the IgM antibodies of the mother cannot pass the placental barrier.

Late Congenital Syphilis

Congenital syphilis after two years of infection may go into latent syphilis similar to that of acquired syphilis. In view of the absence of apparent clinical manifestations, its diagnosis is always made by the reactive standard and specific serological tests. Hence, the latent congenital syphilis, detected accidentally, may be difficult to differentiate from the acquired latent syphilis, after adolescence.

Many clinical manifestations may be seen in late congenital syphilis, but *Hutchinson's triad* consisting of interstitial keratitis, perceptive deafness and Hutchinson's teeth are cardinal.

Clinical Features (Table 11.2)

Interstitial keratitis: It is one of the most common clinical manifestations of late congenital syphilis. It appears between 4 to 30 years of age. Both eyes are affected one after another, the interval between the two varies from a few weeks to many years. Initially, it is characterized by circumcorneal injection, later the blood vessels extend from the limbus into the deeper layer of the cornea. It is followed by infiltration by the cells, giving a hazy appearance to the cornea, resembling ground glass. In mild cases, these changes can be detected only by slit-lamp or corneal microscope. In some cases, it is seen as a bright pink—*salmon patch.* The patient usually presents with impairment of vision, pain, photophobia and watering of the eyes. The symptoms may get aggravated because of associated iridocyclitis. In later stages of the disease the comeal vessels in its deeper layer may remain empty and scarred-ghost vessels and may present as corneal opacities. It is considered to be a hypersensitivity reaction to the treponemes, for it fails to respond to adequate antisyphilitic treatment.

Ears: The internal ear may be affected resulting in progressive perceptive deafness, because of involvement of the cochlear part of the eighth nerve. It is also believed to be a hypersensitivity reaction to the treponemes as it fails to respond to adequate antisyphilitic treatment.

It may be associated with conductive deafness, because of recurrent low grade otitis media.

Hutchinson's teeth: The permanent incisor tooth buds may either be affected in the later part of the pregnancy or in infancy. The central incisors are wide apart, smaller in size with a semilunar notch at its sharp edge, and converging sides like a peg. The notch may appear later because of erosion of deficient enamel. The lateral incisors may similarly be affected (Fig 11.5).

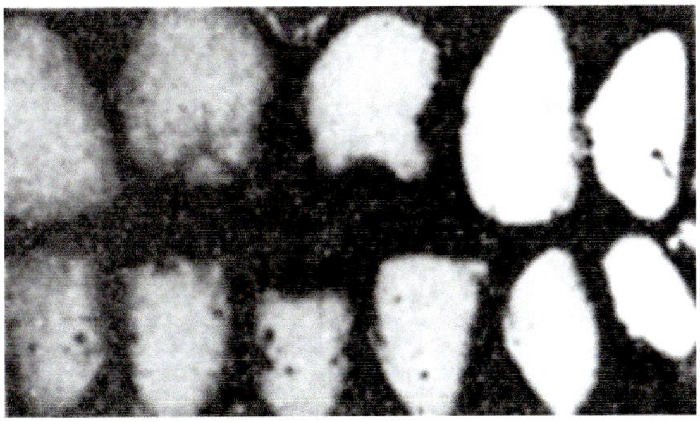

Fig. 11.5: Congenital syphilis, Hutchinson's teeth, central incisors are wide apart with semilunar notch at its sharp edge and a converging sides like a peg (*Courtesy*: Dr OP Homstein and Dr RJ Goriin. The CV Mosby Co, USA)

Gumma

Clinical Features

The gummas may also be the presenting features. They may affect the skin, the mucous membranes, the bones, and the viscera.

Skin and mucous membranes: The gummas may manifest in the form of nodules, noduloulcerative and subcutaneous lesions. The morphological features are similar to that seen in acquired syphilis. Similar type of lesions may be seen on the mucous membranes. Perforations of the palate and the nasopharynx are seen as a common outcome of the gummatous lesions (Fig. 11.6).

Bones and joints: The gummas may involve the long or flat bones. They usually affect the rapidly growing bones like tibia, lower end of the radius and upper end of the ulna, the most common being tibia. They manifest as gummatous osteoperiostitis which may be diffused or localized. The bone is thickened and tender. It may show anterior bowing described as sabre-tibia. Similar situations may occur during infancy. The osteoperiostitis may affect the forehead forming bony swellings—*Parrot's nodes.* The joints may also be affected, causing *syphilitic synovitis.* The patient may present with a painless swelling, with partial restriction of the movements of the joints—*Clutton's joints.* The swelling is due to effusion. Usually, the knee joints are affected. Radiological examination reveals only an increase in the joint space.

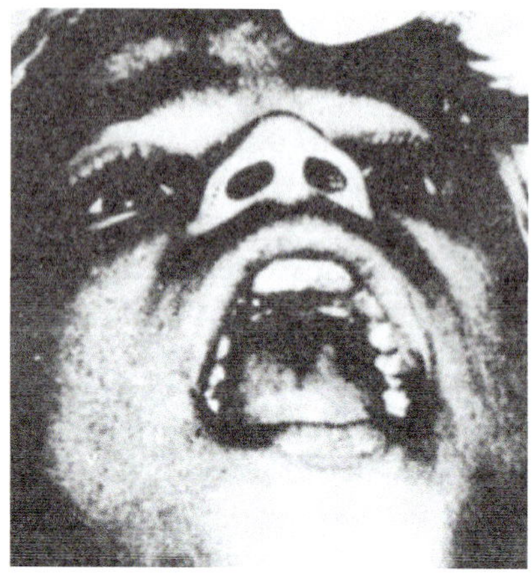

Fig. 11.6: Congenital syphilis. Perforation of the palate

Viscera: The internal organs such as liver, spleen, gastro-intestinal system and testes may show gummatous lesions. The involvement may be asymptomatic or symptoms and signs suggestive of involvement of the respective organs may be present.

Nervous System

The involvement of nervous system is similar to that of acquired syphilis, but at a relatively early age. Asymptomatic meningeal and vascular neurosyphilis are rare, but juvenile general paralysis is more common. Juvenile paresis may precede a varying degree of dementia which may be responsible for mental retardation and impairment of memory. Otherwise, the presenting clinical features and CSF findings are similar to that of acquired syphilis (see Table 8.2). Juvenile tabes may also occur, but it has a mild course. It may be associated with optic atrophy.

Cardiovascular System It is rarely affected.

Paroxysmal Cold Hemoglobinuria

Paroxysmal cold hemoglobinuria is a rare manifestation of late congenital syphilis as well as acquired syphilis. It occurs after exposure to cold. The presenting features may be fever, malaise, backache and passing of port-wine colored urine. The color is due to the presence of hemoglobin, methemoglobin, or RBCs and casts. It occurs in attacks and may be associated with secondary anemia. It is attributed to the presence of hemolysin, which can hemolyze the red blood cells on exposure to cold. Antisyphilitic treatment usually cures it.

Stigmata

These are inactive aftermath, deformities or scars left over by the lesions of early and late congenital syphilis.

Early Stigmata

Syphilitic facies: Characterized by syphilitic rhagades, saddle nose, small maxillae, high arched palate with normal growth of the mandible—*bulldog jaw.*

Teeth The first molar may show a dome-shaped convexity at its free surface called *Moon's molar.* They are prone to get caries. The deformities of the incisor teeth have already been described under

Hutchinson's triad. *Syphilitic onychia* and loss of hair may also be seen. The examination of the eye may reveal a *pepper* and *salt fundus*, characterized by alternate pale atrophic areas surrounded by hyperpigmentation (Table 11.3).

Table 11.3: Early stigmata

1. Facial disfigurement characterized by saddle nose and bulldog jaw
2. Small, widely spaced incisors, with converging sides and notched cutting edge (Hutchison's teeth) *per se* or a part of Hutchison's triad (interstitial keratitis, perceptive deafness, and Hutchison's teeth)
3. Other early stigmata: Rhagades, salt and pepper fundus, and syphilitic onychia.

Late Stigmata

They may be observed over the skin and the mucous membranes in the form of 'tissue paper-scars', deformities and perforation of the palate and the nasopharynx. Optic atrophy and ghost vessels in the cornea may be seen. Perceptive deafness and various deformities of the bone like Parrot's nodes, craniotabes and sabre-tibia are other stigmata (Table 11.4).

Diagnosis It is made by the cardinal clinical manifestations of Hutchinson's triad, and early and late stigmata. The history of maternal syphilis and congenital syphilis may be complementary. The reactive standard and specific serological tests are helpful in the diagnosis. Radiological examination of the affected bones is contributory. CSF examination is essential in cases of asymptomatic and symptomatic neuro-syphilis, the details of which are mentioned in neurosyphilis (see Table 10.2).

Treatment Treatment of congenital syphilis can be divided into prenatal and that of manifest congenital syphilis.

Prenatal Syphilis Congenital syphilis in an infant can be prevented by treating the syphilitic pregnant women. It is envisaged by effective routine antenatal check-up, comprising standard serological tests for syphilis. If active serology is revealed at any stage of pregnancy, adequate specific therapy is warranted for the pregnant mother, with the recommended dosage of penicillin as for acquired syphilis. Furthermore, a rigid follow-up for two years is required for the mother as well as the newborn. In penicillin—sensitive pregnant women, erythromycin may be preferred. Tetracyclines should not be given to them, because of their adverse effects on the bones and the teeth of the infant.

Table 11.4: Stigmata of late lesions

1. Ghost vessels extending from sclera to deep layers of cornea
2. Primary optic atrophy
3. Crushed tissue paper gummatous scars
4. Healed gummatous osteoperiostitis, 'Sabre shin'
5. Incurvature of vertebral borders of scapula
6. Increased carrying angle of forearm
7. Ulnar deviation of middle finger
8. A very short little finger (Dubois sign)

Manifest Congenital Syphilis Penicillin is the drug of choice for the treatment of early as well as late congenital syphilis. Essentially the principles of treatment are the same as for acquired syphilis. It is, however, imperative to calculate the required dosage in individual cases. It is preferable to use procaine/crystalline penicillin (Crys-4, PPF-4, Fortified procaine, penicillin). It is important to bear in mind that with early diagnosis and prompt treatment, the clinical and serological prognosis is better. The CDC recommendations are summarized in Table 11.5.

Late congenital syphilis may be managed according to the schedule for acquired syphilis.

Follow-up

It is carried out in a similar fashion as for early and late syphilis. During the follow-up period if a rising titer of quantitative STS is observed, a repeat course of treatment must be given, even though earlier, an adequate therapy was received by the infant, before or after birth.

Recent World Health Organization (WHO) guidelines for the treatment are included in Table 11.6 as an update for practice wherever indicated

Table 11.5: Congenital syphilis: CDC recommendations

Treatment	Alternatives
1. 100,000-150,000 U/kg of either aqueous procaine penicillin/crystalline penicillin G, 1/M, daily for 10-14 days	NIL

Asymptomatic, seroreactive infante, with normal CSP, born to mothers adequately treated tor syphilis, with penicillin, may be tollowed up for decreasing antibody titers. If titers remain high, treat with benzathine penicillin 50, 000 unite per kg, 1/M, single dose.

Table 11.6: Congenital syphilis treatment: WHO guidelines

Early Congenital Syphilis (Upto 2 years of age)

And infant with abnormal CSF

Recommended regimen

Aqueous benzylpenicillin 1,00000-1 50,000 IU/kg/day administered as 50,000 IU/kg/dose IV every 12 hours during the first 7 days of life every 8 hours and thereafter for a total of 10 days.

Or

Procaine benzylpenicillin 50,000IUkg/day, as a single injection intramuscular, daily for 10 days.

Note: Some experts treat all infants as if the CSF findings were abnormal. Antimicrobials other than penicillin (e.g. erythromycin) are not recommended in young infants except in case of penicillin allergy. Tetracyclines should not be used in young children.

Congrnital syphilis of 2 or more years

Recommended regimen

Aqueous benzylpenicillin 2,00,000-3,00,000 IU/kg/day by intramuscular or intravenous route, administered as 50,000IU /kg/dose every 4-6 hours for 10-14 days

Alternative regimens for penicillin allergic patients, after the first month of life

Erythromucin 7.5-12.5 mg/kg orally 4 times daily for 30 days.

FURTHER READING

1. Darville T. Syphilis. Pediatr Rev 1999;20:160-4.
2. Ewing CI, Roberts C, Davidson DC, Arya OP. Early congenital syphilis still occur. Arch Dis Child 1985;60:1128-33.
3. Fames SW, Setness PA. Serologic tests for syphilis. Postgrad Med 1990;87:37-41.
4. Hollier LM, Cox SM. Syphilis. Semin Perinatol 1998;22:323-31.
5. Wendel GD Jr. Early and congenital syphilis. Obstet Gynecl Clin North Am 1989;16:479-94.
6. Wicher V, Wicher K. Pathogenesis of maternal-fetal syphilis revisited. Clin Infect Dis 2001; 33:354-63.

Chapter 12

Serological Tests for Syphilis

In response to the treponemal infection, three different types of antibodies are produced in the serum namely, reagin, specific antibodies and group-specific antibodies. These antibodies can be demonstrated in the serum of the subjects suffering from syphilis by various serological tests, developed and introduced from time-to-time. They are broadly classified into standard and specific serological tests. The former demonstrates the presence of reagin, while the later the specific and group-specific antibodies.

STANDARD TESTS FOR SYPHILIS

Standard tests for syphilis (STS) are of two types, flocculation (precipitation) and complement-fixation tests. They are based on demonstrating the presence of reagin—a component of IgG and IgM—a substance possessing the properties of an antibody, in individuals suffering from certain diseases including syphilis. The reagin has the capacity to fix the complement and/or form floccules with the colloidal suspension of lipids, extracted from animal tissues. These processes are described as complement fixation and flocculation respectively.

Flocculation Tests

Many tests have been used namely Kahn, Kline, Price, Mazzini, venereal diseases research laboratory (VDRL) test, using either crude lipoidal extracts or 'its synthetic modifications.

At present VDRL is widely used both as a qualitative and quantitative test for the diagnosis of syphilis. This test is easy to perform and has better *sensitivity* and *specificity* than the other flocculation tests.

The VDRL test is performed by adding cardiolipin antigen to the inactivated (heating the serum at 56°C for 30 minutes to remove the complement) serum in tube/slide and rotating mechanically for 4-5 minutes in order to facilitate the formation of floccules. Similarly, quantitative tests are performed on serial dilutions of serum. The test is reactive (positive) when the aggregates of antigen-antibody complexes are noted under the microscope.

Complement-Fixation Tests

The classical Wassermann reaction (WR) has undergone several modifications since its inception. The outlines of the procedure are as follows:

Initially, a measured quantity of antigen (Cardiolipin, cholesterol, lecithin) and complement obtained from guinea pigs's serum, are added to the inactivated serum of an infected subject. The material is incubated at 37°C for 30 minutes. An indicator system comprising the washed sheep's RBCs and serum from rabbit sensitized to sheep's RBCs are added and incubated. The positivity of the test is indicated by absence of hemolysis and vice versa. The control is simultaneously run, wherein saline replaces the serum (Table 12.1).

Table 12.1: Standard tests for syphilis

1. Detect reagins, gammaglobulin fractions that appear in the sera of syphilitics
2. May either be complement fixation tests—Wasserman reactionn (WR), or flocculation tests—VDRL, RPR, Kline, Kahn, Mazzini and Price's precipitation test, automated reagin test, TRUST
3. VDRL reliable and simple may either be qualitative/quantitative; Most widely used screening test
   - Becomes positive 5-6 weeks after infection/2-3 weeks after the appearance of chancre
   - Titres of 1:8 and above diagnostic of syphilis
   - Decreases 4-fold at 3 months, eight-fold at 6 months and returns to normal in 6-12 months after treatment of primary and 12-18 months of secondary syphilis
   - Reactivity may persist despite treatment in late syphilis.

Specific Serological Tests

Many different specific tests have been introduced using antigens obtained from pathogenic (Nichol's strain) or non-pathogenic (Reiter's strain) treponeme, each test detecting different type of antibodies.

In *Treponema pallidum immobilization* (TPI) test, the patient's serum along with the complement are added to a suspension of virulent live *Treponema pallidum* (Nichol's strain) and incubated for 30 minutes. The percentage of organisms immobilized due to the presence of immobilizing antibody in the serum is counted microscopically. The test is considered positive, if more than 50 per cent of the organisms are immobilized.

In the fluorescent treponemal antibody test (FTA), an indirect fluorescent technique is used. The suspected serum is added to a dried smear of Nichol's strain and incubated. If the antibody is present in the serum it will adhere to the treponemes. If fluorescein tagged anti-human globulin is now added and incubated further, the slide will show fluorescence under the ultraviolet microscope. The test detects both the specific and group-specific antibodies. To overcome this difficulty the group-antibodies are first removed from the serum by absorbing and then performing the test, a modification called fluorescent treponemal antibody absorption (FTA-ABS) test. The sorbent used for the absorption being heated culture filtrate of Reiter's treponemes.

Reiter's complement fixation (RCF) and Reiter's protein complement-fixation (RPCF) tests, use the complement-fixation technique, for detecting group-specific antibodies. Here Reiter's strain or its extract is used for performing these tests.

Treponema pallidum Hemagglutination (TPHA) test is popular for routine serodiagnosis of syphilis. It is simple, economical and almost as specific and sensitive as TPI and FTA-ABS tests (Table 12.2).

Many other tests such as *Treponema pallidum* complement fixation (TPCF), whole body treponema complement-fixation (WBTPCF) tests, *Treponema pallidum* immune adherence (TPIA) test, etc. were devised, but have soon fallen into disrepute.

Table 12.2: Specific serological test

1. Detect specific antibodies to the treponemes.
2. TPI
   - Most specific test (100%)
   - Becomes positive, in late primary stage, after reagin tests
   - Seroconversion, only after treatment in early syphilis; tends to remain positive, irrespective of treatment in the late stage
   - Helps to diagnose cardiovascular syphilis (reagin tests may have become nonreactive)
   - Helps to distinguish biological false positive (BPP) from genuine positive
   - Expensive and complicated: not performed routinely
3. FTA-ABS
   - Most sensitive test
   - First to become positive in early syphilis; useful in diagnosis of primary syphilis, before reagins become reactive
   - IgM and 19s IgM FTA-ABS help to distinguish active congenital syphilis from passive maternal transfer of AB
   - Remains positive, inspite of treatment in late syphilis
4. TPHA
   - High specificity and sensitivity intermediate between TPI and FTA-ABS
   - Becomes positive after reagins but before TPI in primary syphilis
   - Inexpensive, reproducible, quantitative and easy to perform
   - May remain positive inspite of treatment in late syphilis
   - MHA-TP is its microvariant
5. RPCF
   - Detects group specific antibodies
   - Not routinely used
6. HATTS

Rapid screening tests These tests were developed for rapid and economical survey of population for syphilis. Standard as well as specific tests have been modified so that they can be performed cheaply within a short-time, specially using automation.

Behavior of Serological Tests

Untreated syphilis: The FTA, test is first to become positive in early syphilis, followed by RPCF and TPHA flocculation and complement-fixation tests. The FTA test, in particular, therefore, is of value in diagnosing these cases of early syphilis, where the demonstration of *Treponema pallidum* is difficult. It is worthwhile to record that reagin starts appearing early in the serum, but the standard test becomes positive only after 15 days of the appearance of primary chancre. The reagin titre, however, continues to rise gradually to reach the maximum in the course of six to eight weeks, which may remain for a period of two years. Subsequently, the titre shows a decline or complete disappearance in late syphilis. TPI test becomes positive later than the other tests *(vide supra)* in early syphilis and may continue to be so throughout life.

Treated syphilis Adequate specific treatment is imperative, for it assists in lowering the titre of reagin, which usually takes four to six months to disappear in early syphilis. But, it may take longer to disappear or may remain positive in lower titres in late syphilis. Fluorescent treponemal antibody (FTA) tests, TPI and others may remain positive throughout life, unless treatment is instituted in the early stages of infection.

Evaluation of the Serological Tests

Standard serological test: The positive standard tests are almost confirmatory, should an affirmative history and clinical evidence of syphilis be present, especially in rising titre and also in high dilutions

(1:8 and above). In view of their cheapness and easy execution furthered by their role in evaluating the prognosis of syphilis after treatment, they score over the other tests. Nevertheless, false positive reactions impose limitations to their use.

Specific tests In latent syphilis and to exclude biological false positive (BFP) reactions they are of immense value. They do not offer any advantage over the standard serological tests so far as the diagnosis of early syphilis is concerned. In late syphilis, however, they are only of confirmatory value. Furthermore they are uneconomical, difficult to perform and have a limited scope in the evaluation of prognosis of syphilis.

The standard as well as the specific serological tests cannot distinguish between syphilis, yaws and other treponematoses.

Hence, the standard serological tests are the mainstay in the routine diagnosis of syphilis in India and in other developing and under developed countries. Specific tests occupy only an ancillary position.

False-positive reactions They are at times encountered as a pitfall of standard serological tests. They are either due to technical errors or biological false-positive (BFP) reactions. The former can easily be obviated by repeating the test, and following the techniques rigidly. The biological false positive (BFP) reactions, on the other hand, are due to formation of a small quantity of reagin in the serum in conditions other than the treponematoses. They manifest either as acute or chronic biological false positive.

Acute biological false-positive (BFP) They are usually transitory and last up to a period of six months. They are commonly seen in acute infections, vaccination and inoculations.

Chronic biological false positive (BFP) They are observed in old age, pregnancy, sometimes in normal individuals and also in chronic infections like leprosy and autoimmune disease.

FURTHER READING

1. Clyne B, Jerrard DA. Syphilis testing. J Emerg Med 2000;18:361-7.
2. Larsen SA, Farshy CE, Pender BJ, Adams MR, Pettit DE, Hambie EA. Staining intensities in the fluorescent treponemal antibody-absorption (FTA-Abs) test association with the diagnosis of syphilis. Sex Transm Dis 1986;13: 221-7.
3. Luger AFM. Serological diagnosis of syphilis: Current methods. In Young H, Mcmillan A (Eds): Immunological Diagnosis of Sexually Transmitted Diseases. New York: Percel Dekker 1988.
4. Miller JN. Value and limitations of non-treponemal and treponemal tests in the laboratory diagnosis of syphilis. Clin Obstet Gynecol 1975;18:191-203.
5. Pangborn MC. A new serologically active phospholipid from beef heart. Proc Soc Exp Biol Med 1941;49:484-6.
6. Rein MF, Banks GW, Logan LC, Larsen SA, Feeley JC, Kellogg DS, et al: Failure of Treponema pallidum immobilization test to provide additional diagnostic information about contemporary problem sera. Sex Transm Dis 1980;7:101-5.

Chapter 13

Chancroid

Chancroid is a sexually transmitted disease caused by *Haemophilus ducreyi,* characterized by multiple, tender, non-indurated, dirty, necrotic genital ulcers with or without suppuration of the inguinal lymph glands.

EPIDEMIOLOGY

It is encountered mainly in the tropics and subtropics. Occasional cases are reported from the other regions. In India, it is found all over the country, at places being the most common STD. It commonly affects individuals with poor hygienic habits, majority of whom belong to the poorer sections of the society. Prostitutes are chiefly responsible for the transmission of the disease. The males are affected more than the females. It usually affects subjects of 20 to 40 years.

ETIOLOGY

The disease is caused by *Haemophilus ducreyi.* It is a gram-negative, short, slender organism with rounded ends. It is 1-2 μ in length and 0.5 μ in width. It is seen in pairs or short chains and 'school of fish' arrangements (Fig. 13.1).

The organism requires enriched media for its culture *in vitro*. It can be grown on a medium containing agar, cystine, dextrose and defibririated rabbit's serum incubated at 35°C.

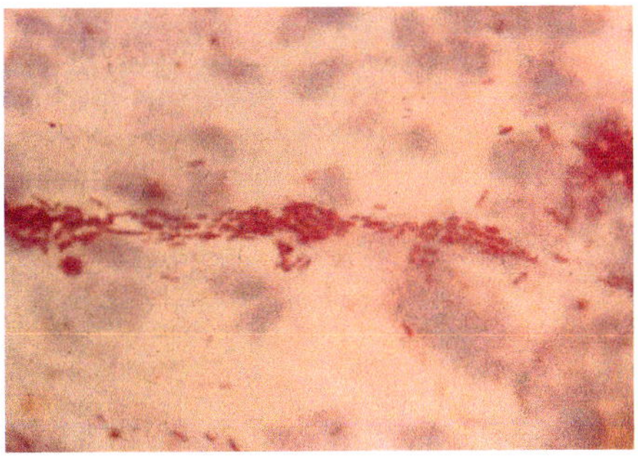

Fig. 13.1: *Haemophilus ducreyi*: 'School of fish' arrangement

PATHOGENESIS

The disease is largely contracted by sexual contact with an infected individual. The organism enters the skin or the mucous membrane of its new host and incites a local tissue reaction. After the requisite incubation period, an erythematous papule appears at the site of inoculation, which soon turns into a pustule, undergoes central necrosis, and forms the characteristic dirty, tender, non-indurated ulcer with undermined edges. Simultaneously, the infection spreads to the surrounding area by autoinoculation and to the regional lymph nodes via the lymphatics. The lymph nodes are inflamed in the initial stage, get matted, and form a unilocular bubo. Later it may suppurate and rupture spontaneously leaving a single discharging sinus.

The histology of the ulcerative lesions often shows certain constant features. The space below the floor of the ulcer can be arbitrarily divided into three zones, the superficial zone, mid zone and deeper zone. The superficial zone is seen to consist of necrotic tissue and an acute inflammatory infiltrate. The mid zone is much broader and contains the new blood vessels showing patchy proliferative changes on the one hand, and degenerative changes on the other. The deeper zone shows a chronic inflammatory infiltrate comprising plasma cells and lymphocytes.

INCUBATION PERIOD

It is usually from one to five days. Occasionally, it may be longer.

CLINICAL FEATURES

The characteristic lesions are multiple, small superficial, painful, dirty, necrotic ulcers situated on the genitals (Figs 13.2A and B). Occasionally, a single lesion is observed. The ulcers are of varying shapes and sizes. The edges of the lesions are undermined and surrounded by a narrow zone of erythema and edema. The floor is covered by dirty necrotic tissue. The lesions are non-indurated, tender and bleed on touch. A purulent discharge is usually present. There may be an inguinal bubo at the same time (Figs 13. 3A and B).

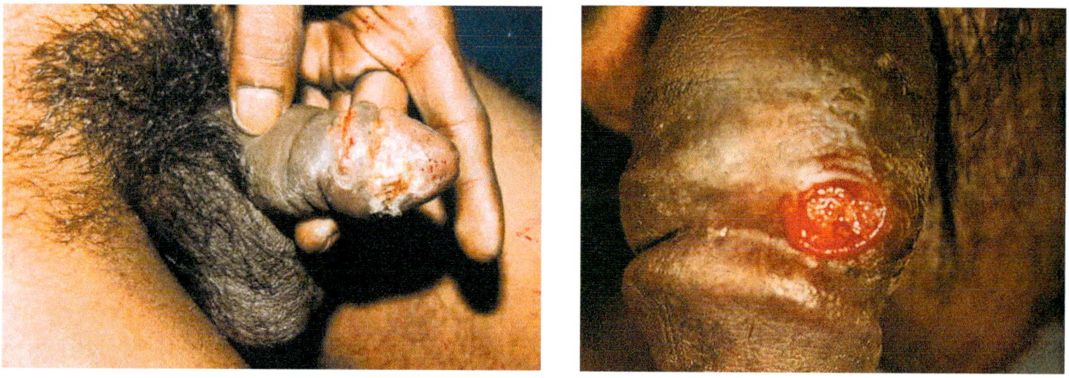

Figs 13.2A and B: Chancroid. Multiple superficial dirty necrotic ulcers on the preputial orifice

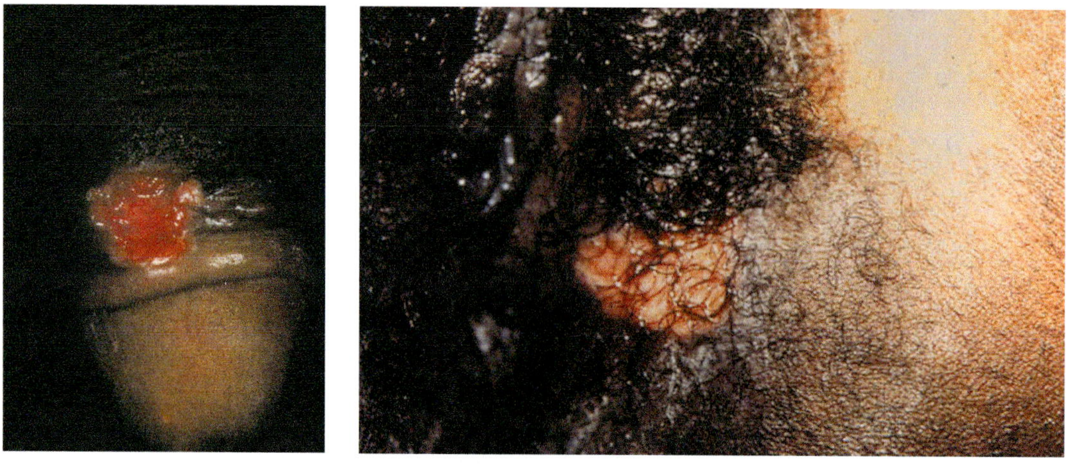

Figs 13.3A and B: Chancroid. A single ulcer with burst bubo

It presents usually as a unilateral, unilocular tender swelling. The surface is taut and erythematous in the earlier stages. In the later stages, there is fluctuation (Fig 13.4). Sometimes a burning sensation during micturition is present, if the urine flows over the ulcer. Occasionally, malaise and fever are experienced by some patients.

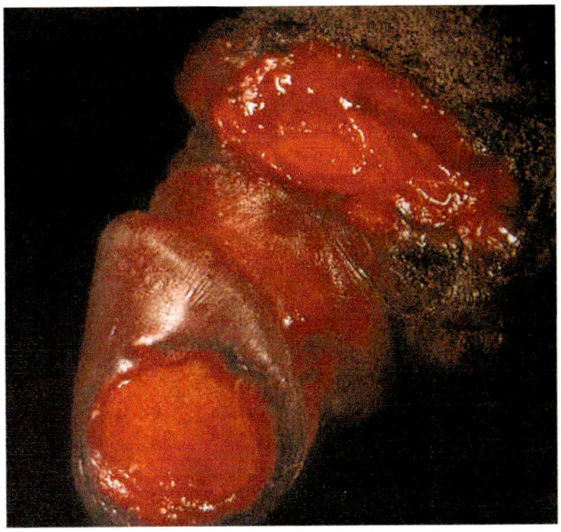

Fig. 13.4: Chancroid unilateral bubo

Variants

At times chancroid may show variations as described below.

- *Dwarf chancroid*: It is characterized by a small superficial ulceration (Fig 13.5).
- *Giant chancroid:* It is a large granulomatous ulcer, secondary to a ruptured bubo extending on to the surrounding parts.
- *Follicular chancroid:* These lesions are seen in association with the hair follicles, specially in women and simulate folliculitis in the early stages, but later breakdown to form ulcers.
- *Transient chancroid:* The lesions are very superficial and exist only for a short-time, followed by the classical inguinal bubo.
- *Serpiginous chancroid:* It is characterized by multiple ulcers, coalescing to form a serpiginous pattern.
- *Mixed infection*: Sometimes chancroid is associated with primary chancre.

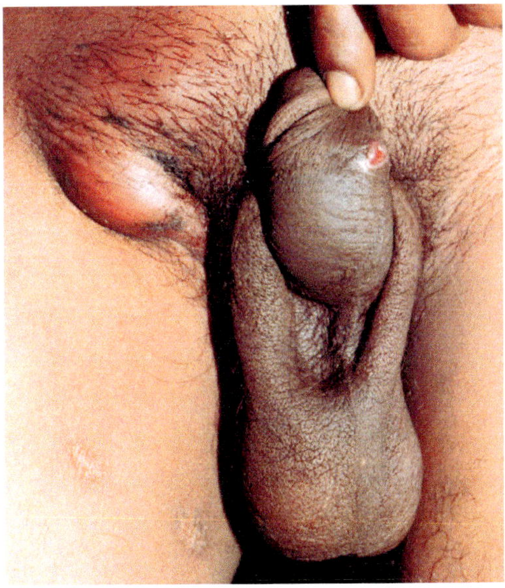

Fig. 13.5: Dwarf chancroid

Sites

Genital: They may occur anywhere on the genitals. In males, they are commonly found on the under surface of the prepuce, preputial orifice and shaft of the penis. The glans penis, coronal sulcus and the frenum are less frequently involved. In females, the lesions are seen chiefly on the labia majora, fourchette, and at times on the labia minora.

Extragenital Chancroid may rarely affect sites other than genital. These sites are the thighs, around the anus, abdomen, hands, breast and mouth.

COURSE

The ulcers may heal in a few days time without any further complications. At other times they may enlarge slowly and become resistant to treatment. The bubo may rupture and heal or leave behind a discharging sinus. Sometimes it may form a giant ulcer. Secondary infection by Vincent's organism may complicate the lesions leading to destructive changes.

COMPLICATIONS

The most common complication is a discharging sinus resulting from a ruptured bubo. The affection of the preputial orifice may give rise to phimosis. Balanoposthitis is quite common in the acute stage. Paraphimosis is sometimes seen. Phagedenic changes and fistulae may occur. Massive bouts of bleeding can take place, if a blood vessel gets involved in the destructive process (Table 13.1).

DIAGNOSIS

It is based on history of sexual exposure with an infected person, a short incubation period and the characteristic morphology of the lesion.

Other genital ulcers such as syphilitic chancre, herpes progenitalis, granuloma inguinale, lymphogranuloma venereum and traumatic ulcers need be differentiated from chancroid by appropriate clinical features and laboratory methods. It is confirmed by the demonstration of the organism from smears prepared from a clean ulcer or an aspirate from a bubo. The smears are stained either by Gram's or Pappenheim's stain. It may, however, be difficult to demonstrate the organisms.

Further, the confirmation of the diagnosis may be made by the culture of the organism in an enriched medium, intradermal test and histopathology.

Intradermal test or Ito-Reenstierna test becomes positive one to two weeks after the appearance of the sore and remains positive throughout the life. The test is performed by injecting 0.1 ml of the suspension of the killed organisms intradermally while 0.1 ml of normal saline serves as control on the contralateral site. The test is inferred as positive only when a nodule of 5 mm or more in diameter appears at the test site after 24 hours. This test is not routinely performed and is only of academic interest. Histology of the lesions may complement the clinical diagnosis.

Table 13.1: Chancroid

1. Multiple, small, superficial, painful, dirty necrotic ulcers; base is nonindurated and edges are undermined; tender and bleed on touch
2. A unilateral, unilocular, tender inguinal bubo
3. Ulcers are either classical, or dwarf, giant, follicular, transient, phagedenic, chancroidal
4. Undersurface of prepuce, preputial orifice, shaft of penis are the site in man; labia majora, minora and fourchette are affected in women
5. Ruptured bubo, balanoposthitis, phimosis, paraphimosis may complicate chancroid.

TREATMENT

Erythromycin and Ceftriaxone are the drugs of choice. The details of treatment are outlined in Table 13.2.

Table 13.2: Chancroid treatment recommended schedule

Drug	*Dosage*	*Status*
1. Erythromycin	500 mg, 4 times a day for 7 days	Treatment of choice
2. Ceftriaxone	250 mg I/M, single dose	Effective and treatment of choice
3. Trimethoprim/Sulfamethoxazole	160/800 mg, twice a day for 7 days	Increasing resistance
4. Amoxycillin + Clavalanic acid	500 mg + 125 mg thrice a day for 7 days	

Table 13.3: Chancroid treatment: WHO guidelines

Recommended regimens
Ciprofloxacin 500 mg orally twice a day for 3 days
Or Erythromycin base 550 mg orally 4 times a day for 7 days
Or Azithromycin 1 gm, orally as a single dose
Alternative regimen
Ceftriaxone 250 mg, as a single intramuscular injection.

Recent World Health Organization (WHO) guidelines are provided, in addition, in Table 13.3 to facilitate their use for the future.

FURTHER READING

1. Donders GG. Treatment of sexually transmitted bacterial diseases in pregnant women. Drugs 2000; 59: 477-85.
2. Greenblatt RB. Management of chancroid, granuloma inguinale, lymphogranuloma venereum in general practice. US Public Health Service Publication, No. 255, 1953.
3. Lewis DA. Diagnostic tests for chancroid. Sex Transm Infect 2000;76: 137-41.
4. Lewis DA. The use of experimental animal and human models in the study of chancroid pathogenesis. Int J STD AIDS 1999;10:71-79.
5. Schmid GP. Treatment of chancroid, 1997. Clin Infect Dis 1999;28: S14-S20.

Chapter 14

Lymphogranuloma Venereum

INTRODUCTION

Lymphogranuloma venereum is a sexually transmitted disease affecting the lymphatic tissue caused by an organism of the genus *Chlamydia,* characterized by a primary herpetiform genital lesion, followed by suppurative, multiloculated inguinal adenitis and anal syndrome.

EPIDEMIOLOGY

The disease is commonly seen in tropical and subtropical countries, but sporadic cases are known to occur all over the world. In India, it is prevalent in Tamil Nadu and Andhra Pradesh. It affects both men and women, usually in the age group of 20 to 40 years, irrespective of race and religion. It is commonly seen in unhygienic individuals and prostitutes. The prostitutes by and large are responsible for its spread, because it remains occult in them.

ETIOLOGY

The causative organism was identified in 1930 by Wallace and Hellerstrom as a large virus belonging to the psittacosis-lymphogranuloma group. Presently, the organism is included under the genus *Chlamydia.* Its biological nature is still controversial. Man is the only natural host of the organism, but it can be experimentally transmitted to monkeys, guinea-pigs and mice by inoculation. It can also be grown in the chick embryo.

PATHOGENESIS

The organism enters the host through abraded mucous membrane/skin by sexual contact or otherwise. It has got a special predilection for the lymphatic tissue, where it incites an inflammatory response resulting in edema and proliferation of the endothelial lining of the lymphatics. This in turn leads to blockage of regional lymphatics, necrotic ulceration, fibrosis and stricture formation. The pathological changes in the initial herpetic lesion are largely nonspecific. The lymph nodes may, however, show specific changes characterized by stellate abscesses consisting of polymorphonuclear leukocytes and macrophages. They are surrounded by epithelioid cells and chronic granulation tissue containing numerous plasma cells. In the later stages, they may show extensive fibrosis and large areas of caseation necrosis.

INCUBATION PERIOD

It varies from a few days to three weeks, with an average of a week.

CLINICAL FEATURES

Early Manifestations

It starts as a transient painless, non-indurated, herpetiform papule, vesicle or a pustule on the genitals. It may pass off unnoticed. At times it may present as an extensive ulcer or a nodule. Intraurethral lesions may present as nonspecific urethritis.

Site

In males the lesions occur on the coronal sulcus, the urethra and the glans penis, while in females it affects the vulva, the urethra and the posterior vaginal wall.

The constitutional symptoms are variable and are usually associated with early manifestations. They are characterized by malaise, chills, fever, headache and joint pains. The liver and the spleen may also be enlarged.

The secondary lesions appear after a varying period of weeks, months or years. They are recognised as inguinal, urethral, genital, rectal or anorectal syndromes, the latter three occur as late manifestations.

Inguinal Syndrome

It usually manifests after an incubation period of 10 to 90 days. The males are affected more than the females. It is followed by an unilateral, multilocular swelling in the groin. The swelling is firm and elastic. The lymph glands are matted together and are adherent to the overlying skin and subjacent tissues. The skin is thickened and inflamed. The swelling is divided into an upper and lower group of masses by the inguinal ligament and the line of demarcation is described as the 'sign of groove' (Fig. 14.1). The swelling may soften and suppurate, eliciting fluctuation. It opens on the skin surface to form multiple sinuses, discharging seropurulent or purulent material. The swelling may show spontaneous resolution or a chronic stationary indolent mass may persist for a long period. In case the iliac lymph glands are affected, the patients report with pain in the abdomen, which may be mistaken, if on the right side, for appendicitis.

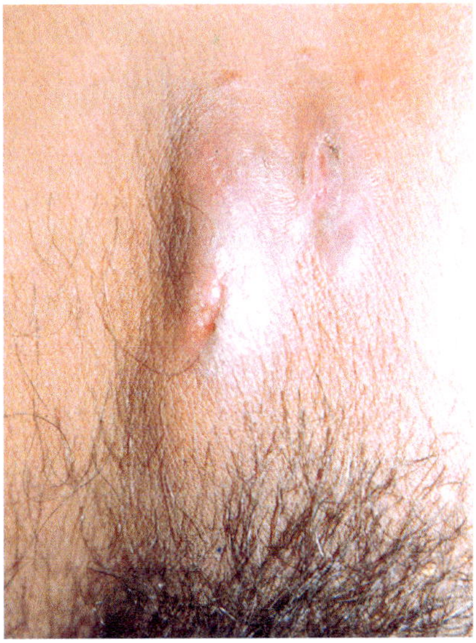

Fig. 14.1: Lymphogranuloma venereum. Swelling above and below the inguinal ligament showing the 'sign of groove'

Late Manifestations

Genital Syndrome

It may appear after a few months or years. The women are affected more than the men. They may occur alone or in association with similar changes in the anus or the rectum. It is due to chronic lymphedema and stasis of the inguinal glands. It manifests in females, as elephantiasis of the vulva and the clitons. The swelling may be localized to one side of the labium or part of the labium. The skin over the swelling is initially smooth, but later becomes warty, verrucose or mammillated. Its size varies from a small to large multilobulated pendulous mass hanging down and barricading the vulval cleft. The ulcers over the swelling are usually chronic and indolent. They are present on the inner surface of labia minora, the fourchette, around the urethra and the clitoris (Figs 14.2A and B). At times, urethral and vaginal strictures are also seen. In males, it appears as elephantiasis of the penis and the scrotum. It may also be associated with ulcers (Figs 14.3A and B).

Urethral Syndrome

It is the late feature. Intraurethral lesion, causes urethral stricture and fistula.

Anorectal Syndrome

It appears after a few months or years of infection. It affects both men and women. It is either due to direct spread of infection from the genitals or due to involvement of anorectal or pelvic lymph glands. The condition is asymptomatic or attended by pruritus, and is characterized by perianal edema (proctitis) and edema of the mucous membrane of the rectum. Later multiple perianal fissures appear over the skin. Firm, elastic swellings are also noted under the mucous membrane, which may either be hypertrophic pararectal tissue or infected anorectal or pararectal lymph glands. These swellings

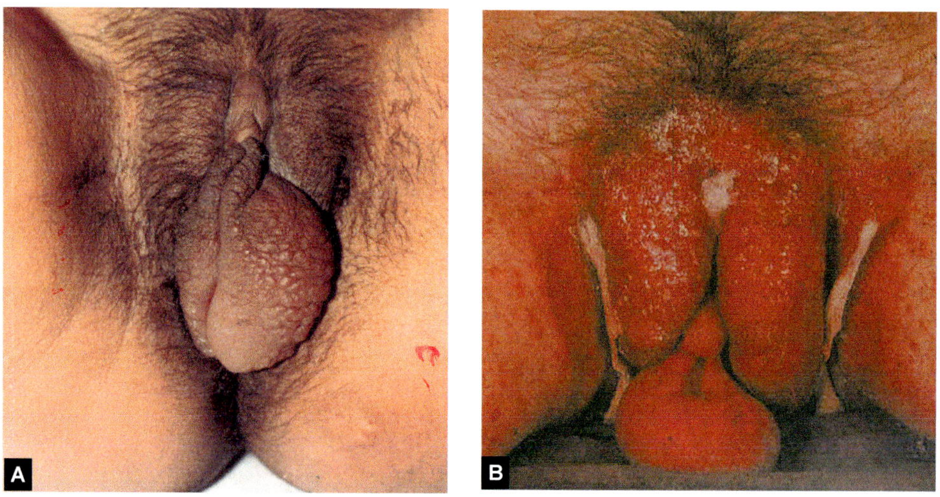

Figs 14.2A and B: Lymphogranuloma venereum. Esthiomene of the clitoris

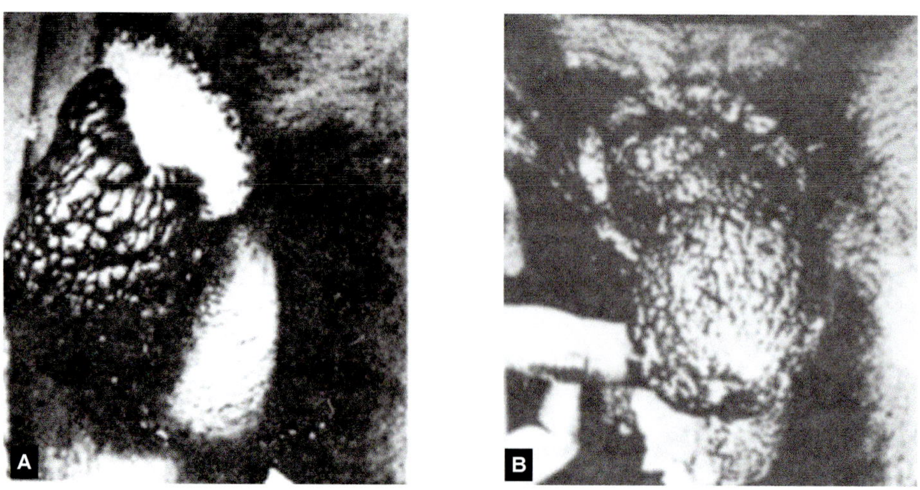

Figs 14.3A and B: Lymphogranuloma venereum. Elephantiasis of the penis

may suppurate and burst into the rectum or track down to form perianal and ischiorectal abscesses, resulting in multiple fistulae. In an advanced case of this syndrome, the patient reports with long-standing history of rectal pain and tenesmus. There is an increasing difficulty in defecation and discharge of pus streaked with blood per rectum. The attacks of constipation may alternate with diarrhea. Per-rectum examination may reveal a stricture of the rectum. Nodules and ulcers of the mucous membrane of the rectum are also found. Rectal polyps simulating hemorrhoids may occur. Carcinoma of the rectum is a sequel of the disease (Table 14.1).

Table 14.1: Lymphogranuloma venereum

Early manifestations

1. Transient, painless, asymptomatic, self-healing, non-indurated, herpetiform papule, populovesicle/pustule on genitals
2. Inguinal syndrome
   - Manifests after an incubation period of 10-90 days
   - Enlarged lymph nodes form a firm, elastic unilateral, multilocular swelling in inguinal region; *Sign of groove*, is cardinal
   - May open on the surface through multiple sinuses/undergo spontaneous resolution
3. Climatic bubo
   - Enlargement of femoral group of lymph nodes
4. Bubonuli and seaphone penis

Late manifestations

1. Genital syndrome
   - Appears after a few months/years
   - 'Esthiomene', (elephantiasis of the vulva) clitoris, labia; warty verrucuous growths and indolent chronic ulcers may complicate
   - Similar changes, uncommonly affect male genitalia
2. Anorectal syndrome
   - Appears after a few months/years
   - Results either from direct affliction/involvement of anorectal and pelvic group of lymph nodes
   - Proctitis, anorectal strictures, perianal, ischiorectal abscesses, and fistulae are cardinal
   - Carcinoma may be a sequela

Diagnosis

It is suspected by the history of occurrence of a herpetiform lesion on the genitals, a few days after the sexual intercourse, followed by painful unilateral, multilocular inguinal bubo. The other ulcerative conditions namely *chancroid, syphilis, herpes progenitalis,* and *granuloma* inguinale, with/without inguinal bubo should be excluded by the characteristic clinical features and appropriate laboratory investigations. Furthermore, conditions like filariasis, tuberculosis, *Hodgkin's disease, infectious mononucleosis, lymphatic leukemia* and *malignancy,* affecting the inguinal glands, should also be ruled out. The diagnosis is confirmed by the following tests.

Culture

The pus is aspirated from an unruptured bubo. It is cultured in the yolk sac of the chick embryo. The organisms isolated from the pure culture are identified.

Frei's (Intradermal) Test

It becomes positive usually two to three weeks after the appearance of the bubo. The test is performed by injecting 0.1 ml of lygranum (a commercially available antigen prepared from the growth of the organisms in the yolk sac of the chick embryo), intradermally into one forearm and 0.1 ml of the contents of normal yolk sac into the other, serving as control. The positivity is indicated by the appearance of a papule of 6 mm or more in diameter with surrounding erythema at the site of injection.

Complement-fixation Test

This is a sensitive and reliable test. The antibodies appear early in the serum, but they attain the maximum level in the three to six weeks after the appearance of the bubo. The test when positive in a dilution of 1:40 and above, is suggestive of infection.

Hypergammaglobulinemia

It is a constant finding in this condition.

Treatment

Tetracyclines are the drugs of choice. The details of treatment outline in Table 14.2. In addition to the above therapy, surgical intervention may be needed in cases with complications like abscesses, fistulae and strictures.

Table 14.2: Treatment of lymphogranuloma venereum

Drug	*Dosage*	*Status*
1. Tetracycline	500 mg, four times a day for 2-3 weeks	Treatment of choice
2. Doxycycline	100 mg, twice a day for 2 weeks	Treatment of choice
3. Erythromycin	500 mg, four times a day for at least 2 weeks	Treatment of choice
4. Sulfamethoxazole	1.0 g orally, twice a day for at least 2 weeks	Alternative

Bubo may be aspirated before it breaks down.

Table 14.3: Lymphogranuloma venereum treatment: WHO guidelines

Recommended regimen

Doxycyclline 100 mg, twice a day for 14 days

Or Erythromycin 500 mg 4 times a day for 14 days

Alternative regimen

Tetracycline 500 mg 4 times a day for 14 days

Note: Tetracyclines are contraindicated in pregnancy

Fluctuant lymph nodes should be aspirated through healthy skin. Incision and drainage or excision of lymph nodes might delay healing. Some patients with advanced diseases might require treatment for longer than 14 days and sequelae such as stricture and fistulae may require surgery.

In addition, recent World Health Organization (WHO) guidelines are also highlighted for the future use in Table 14.3

FURTHER READING

1. Greenblatt RB. Management of chancroid, granuloma inguinale, lymphogranuloma venereum in general practice. US Public Health Service Publication, No 255, 1953.
2. Rajam RV, Rangiah PN. Lymphogranuloma venereum, Monograph Series No. 1, Supplement to Ind J Dermatol Venereal 1955.
3. Faro S. Lymphogranuloma venereum, chancroid, and granuloma inguinale. Obstet Gynecol Clin North Am 1989;16: 517-30.
4. Gupta S, Ajith C, Kanwar AJ, Sehgal VN, Kumar B, Mete U. Genital elephantiasis and sexually transmitted infections—revisited. Int J STD AIDS. 2006; 17: 157-65.

Chapter 15

Granuloma Inguinale

INTRODUCTION

Granuloma inguinale, a mildly contagious, autoinoculable granulomatous condition, was described in 1882 by McLeod as serpiginous ulceration. Its causative organism was recovered from oral lesions by Donovan in 1905, as intracellular protozoans. The organism was subsequently demonstrated in large numbers in large mononuclear cells: However, Aragao and Vianna are credited with naming 'it *Calymmatobacterium granulomatis*. Goidzieher and Peck identified Donovan bodies in histologic sections and narrated the classic clinical description.

The specific histology of granuloma inguinale was described by Pund and Greenblatt, including its pathognomonic name (cell of Greenblatt). Greenblatt *et al* later produced the disease experimentally in volunteers by injecting material from an unruptured bubo and also described 'pseudobubo' formation as its clinical manifestation. A major breakthrough came when Donovan recognized intracellular bodies from an oral lesion of the disease as the incriminated agent. These are now called Donovan bodies. Goidzieher and Peck recognized these bodies in histologic sections of the tissue. Their observations, the first of their kind, helped considerably in alleviating existing doubts. However, their claim of having cultivated an intracellular capsulated bacillus was unconvincing.

DeMonbreun and Goodpasture succeeded in isolating a bacillus of the aerogen group from lesions and feces of patients with granuloma inguinale. They could demonstrate a morphologic resemblance to Donovan bodies in culture, but they failed to transmit the infection to animals. They documented that the disease was a chronic intestinal infection by the aerogen group of bacilli, with secondary fecal contamination of the skin. McIntosh was the first to successfully transmit the disease experimentally. He also had reported that Donovan bodies were the causative organism of the disease and demonstrated changes in agglutinins, serum proteins, and skin sensitivity, suggesting production of antibodies against Donovan bodies.

Until the end of the 1930s, the controversy regarding the nature of the etiologic organism remained unsolved. Greenblatt *et al* were successful in producing granuloma inguinale in three human subjects. They were of the view that the Donovan bodies were sporozoans because of their affinity for mononuclear cells. Histologic examination of lymph nodes revealed Donovan bodies, from which it was surmised that lymphatics could also be affected, Anderson was able to culture *C. granulomatis* on the yolk sac of chick embryos. Later, Anderson *et al* described the process in detail. They inoculated the yolk sac of a chick embryo with contaminant-free tissue from a patient with granuloma inguinale. The first embryo with a positive culture was obtained after 17 days having been inoculated 6 days previously. Serial cultures in 9-, 10-, or 11-day-old embryos produced for the most part unencapsulated organisms. Encapsulated organisms were produced if propagation was done on 4-to 6-day-old chick embryos. On the basis of their successful culture of the organism, they proposed a new genus, *Donovania granulomatis.*

The aforementioned attempts showed that previous so-called cultures of the Donovan microorganism were highly doubtful and were probably not of the organism itself but of contaminants. Encouraged by the culture of *D. granulomatis* on the yolk sac of chick embryo, other investigators tried to discover an artificial medium for cultivation. Only partial success was achieved by Dunham and Rake. Following this, Goldberg *et al* defined and demonstrated the bacteriologic behavior of *D. granulomatis.* Goldberg pointed out that factors such as a low O-R potential, which can be achieved by a thioglycollate medium and a factor (or factors) present in egg, were necessary for the growth of *D. granulomatis.* The egg factor could be substituted by the enzymatic digestion of bovine albumin or soya meal. Goldberg also succeeded in isolating a bacterium resembling *D. granulomatis* from the feces of a patient with granuloma inguinale. Recently, study of basic hematologic profile and lymphocyte subpopulations (T lymphocytes with subsets T4 helper/inducer, T8 suppressor/cytotoxic, and B lymphocytes) showed its general increase. In addition, an overall increase in B-lymphocyte and immunoglobulin levels was also evident. It is envisaged that distribution of T cell subsets and immunoglobulin-synthesizing B lymphocytes in the tissues, and their ultimate correlation with blood findings, may substantially add to further elucidation of the bacterium's natural history.

Granuloma inguinale is now considered a sexually transmitted disease, and its occurrence has been reported from endemic as well as from so-called nonendemic areas. It is characterized by granulomatous ulceration of the genitalia and neighboring sites. It is caused by *Calymmatobacterium granulomatis.*

Some synonyms for granuloma inguinale are donovanosis, granuloma venereum, serpiginous ulcer of the groin, ulcerating granuloma of the pudenda, chronic venereal sore, and granuloma inguinal tropicum.

Granuloma inguinale is endemic in many parts of the world, sporadic in certain places, and rarely epidemic. Presently, the disease is sparingly reported from Europe, Japan, and other temperate zones. China, Jamaica, and some parts of Papua New Guinea have shown a sizable decline in endemicity in the recent past, while in Vietnam, Indonesia, Africa, southern Papua New Guinea, and southern India the disease continues to be endemic. Racial susceptibility, hot and humid climate, low socioeconomic status, lack of personal hygiene, poor educational standards, and sexual promiscuity are all factors in its occurrence and transmission. Generally, prostitutes are the reservoir of the disease.

CLINICAL FEATURES

Onset of the disease is marked by formation of a firm papule. This may erode to form an ulcer, expressed as an ulcerogranulomatous, hypertrophic, sclerotic, or necrotic variant (Table 15.1).

1. *Ulcerative/ulcerogranulomatous variant:* A single well-defined, friable, beefy red, nontender, nonindurated ulcer with profuse granulation tissue, bleeding on touch and showing no necrosis on the surface (Figs 15.1A to C). Atypical variants may be encountered. Secondary infection of the ulcer may cause it to become tender, with necrotic slough and regional lymphadenopathy. Multiple lesions may occasionally be encountered. Ulcers of longer duration have a tendency to spread slowly, leading to the formation of a well-marked, raised margin at the edge of the ulcer. They often exhibit less granulation tissue. Chronicity may result in mild induration.
2. *Hypertrophic:* An irregular, friable raised growth bleeding on touch or an ulcer with a well-defined raised edge and an elevated granulomatous base is the usual presentation (Figs 15.2A and B).

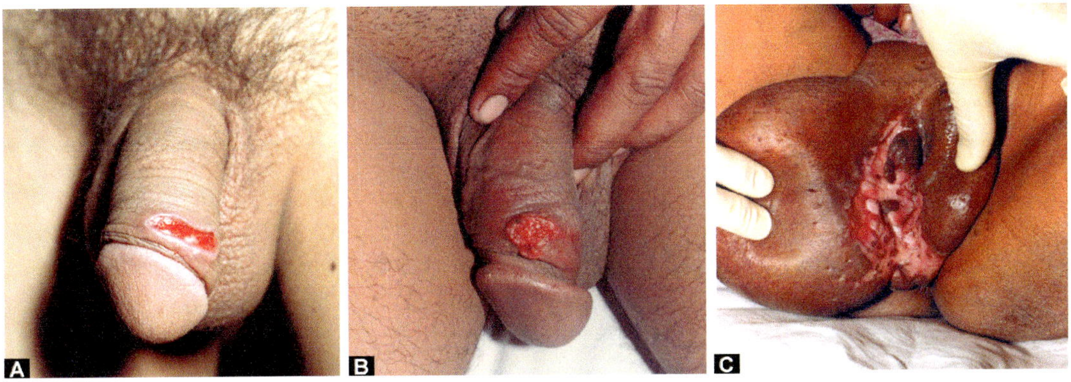

Figs 15.1A to C: A granulomatous ulcer with wavy outline on the shaft of the penis

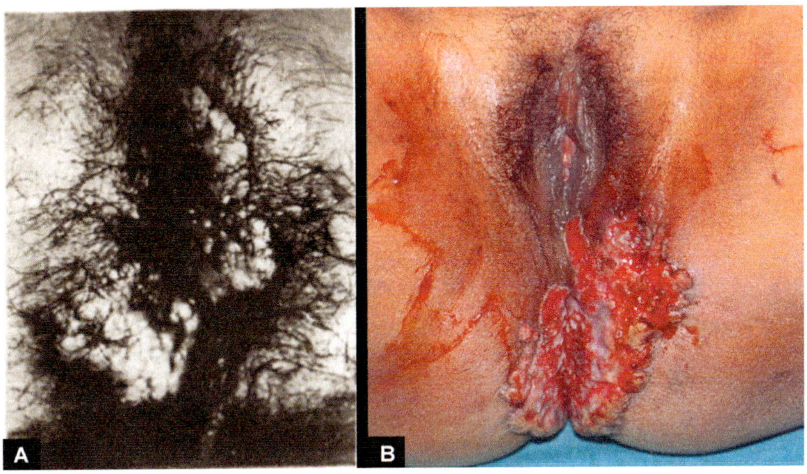

Figs 15.2A and B: Hypertrophic type affecting the perianal region

Table 15.1: Granuloma ingulnale (Donovanosis)

1.	Fleshy, exuberant, beefy-red, non-indurated, nontender, single ulcer with overflowing (everted) edges
2.	Prepuce, coronal sulcus, shaft, glans, and frenulum are common sites in men while in women, it affects labia majora, labia minora, and perianal region
3.	Extragenital sites, are occasionally affected
4.	Ulcerogranulomatous, hypertrophic, necrotic, and sclerotic are the clinical variants
5.	Lymphadenopathy is conspicuously absent
6.	Pseudobubo, swelling of subcutaneous tissue of inguinal region, may be encountered.

3. *Sclerotic:* A deep, nontender, nonindurated ulcer with a clean floor and straight to undermined, non-bleeding edges, with waxing and waning of the activity. Atypical forms may be encountered.
4. *Necrotic: h*A large foul-smelling, tender, non-indurated, irregular ulcer developing rapidly in the course of a few days, resulting in destruction of the genitalia.

A true bubo is generally not formed in granuloma inguinale. Sometimes, however, the subcutaneous tissue of the groin is affected, probably through lymphatics, leading to a fluctuant swelling. This has been named by Greenblatt *et al* a "pseudobubo". This swelling usually ruptures, forming a clean, raised granulomatous ulcer.

The perianal region can be affected following homosexual contact. Dissemination of the disease to other parts of the body, such as the oral cavity, lip, gums, pharynx, cheeks, eyelid, sternum, thorax, abdomen, ribs, clavicles, and colon may also occur.

Metastatic lesions of granuloma inguinale in bones have also been reported. Of the 11 cases of bone disease thus far recorded, 10 were in women with lesions on the cervix. Osteolytic lesions are the usual presentation in the skeletal system.

COMPLICATIONS AND SEQUELAE

The most important sequela of granuloma inguinale, which has been studied quite extensively, is its relationship to squamous cell carcinoma of the penis. Pund and Greenblatt in a histopathologic study of the disease found pronounced epithelial proliferation, simulating early epitheliomatous changes. Beerman and Sonck graded pseudoepitheliomatous hyperplasia seen in the disease into grades I, II, and III. They concluded that when hyperplasia extended deeply enough, a diagnosis of carcinoma of the penis could be made.

Rajam and Rangiah emphasized that the resemblance between granuloma inguinale and carcinoma can be close, on both clinical and histologic grounds. A true epitheliomatous change can occur as a complication or sequela to granuloma inguinale but seems to be an infrequent occurrence.

Besides carcinoma, other complications are adhesions to the scrotum and penis, destruction of the penile shaft, pseudobubo, and pseudoelephantiasis. Stenosis of the urethral, vaginal, or anal orifice is a complication of the sclerotic variety of the disease. Pseudoelephantiasis is an unusual, sparingly reported entity. It occurs in both men and women and is characterized by morphology simulating that of elephantiasis of the genitals (Fig. 15.4). Differentiation from the latter is made on the basis of conspicuous ulcer(s) preceding the swelling and absence of constitutional symptoms of fever, weakness, and arthralgia. Mechanical obstruction of the lymphatics following scarring may cause this condition. Other unusual sites are the gingiva, uterus, fallopian tubes, ovary, buttock, lymph node, and epididymis. Sehgal *et al* presented an extremely rare case of primary extragenital disseminated cutaneous granuloma inguinale.

DIAGNOSIS

The diagnosis of granuloma inguinale may appear simple if 'it is suspected whenever ulcers appear over the genitalia. Confirmation should, however, be through demonstration of Donovan bodies in the tissue smears and also by histopathological examination of the tissue sections.

Donovan bodies are identified in smears as mature and/or immature organisms present inside the cytoplasm of mononuclear cells. These cells may exhibit vacuolation inside the cytoplasm. The mature organism is ovoid or bean-shaped, varying from 1 to 1.5 m in length and 0.5 to 0.7 m in thickness, with a well-defined pinkish material surrounding a blue bacillary body. In addition, it has dark-blue chromatin inclusion arranged at the poles. The capsule may remain unstained or stain bright pink. The morphology of the immature organism may conform to a coccoid, diplococcoid, or bacillary form. The organism varies in size from 0.6 to 1.0 m. The diplococcoid forms in parti-cular are interesting, resembling a closed safety pin (Figs 15.3 and 15.4A to C).

Tissue smears cannot be overemphasized, even though they may be negative in up to one-third of cases ulcerogranulomatous, necrotic, and sclerotic variety. It is thus imperative to perform histopathologic examination of tissue section.

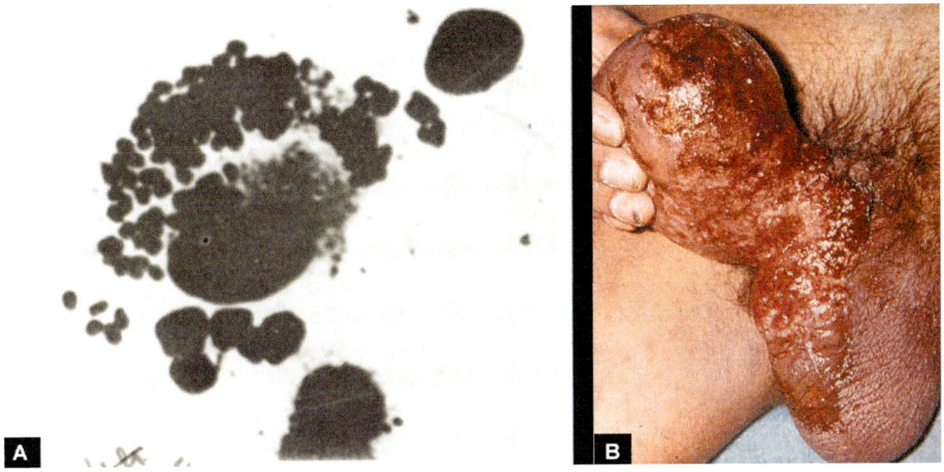

Figs 15.3A and B

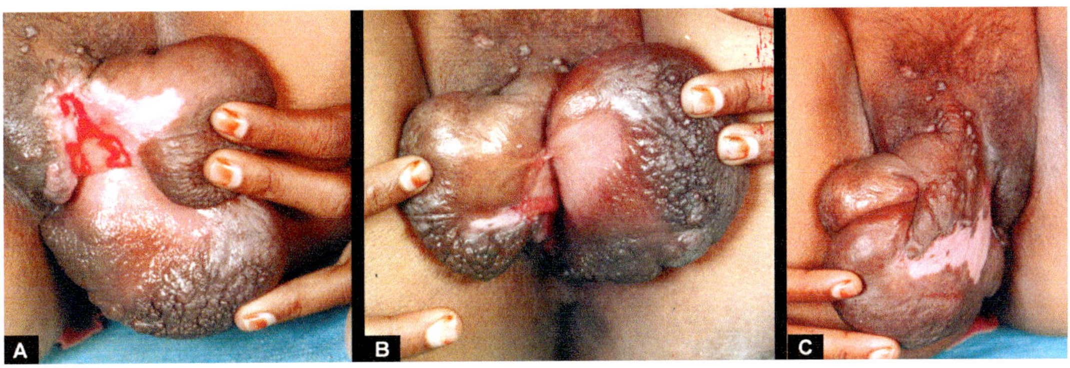

Figs 15.3A and B and 15.4A to C: Elephantiasis of genitals

Initially, it was believed that the histopathologic changes of granuloma inguinale were non-specific, and not sufficiently characteristic to permit a diagnosis on tissue section. Pund and Greenblatt indicated, however, that a massive cellular reaction surch arged with plasma cells, a paucity of lymphocytes, a diffuse sprinkling as well as focal collections of polymorphs in papillae, pseudoepitheliomatous changes, and pathognomonic mononuclear cells filled with intracytoplasmic cysts containing darkly staining bodies were unique enough to make the diagnosis. Recently, Sehgal *et al* have emphasized the distinctive histopathologic features that affect the dermis as well as the epidermis.

The dermal changes are primarily inflammatory. They consist of a dense infiltrate, formed predominantly of large numbers of plasma and mononuclear cells throughout the dermis (Figs 15.5 to 15.7). In addition, histiocytes are seen in varying numbers.

A few large cells containing cystic spaces, often with nuclei pushed to one side, and darkly staining inclusions (cells of Greenblatt) are conspicuous. The number of neutrophils and lymphocytes is insignificant in most sections. Donovan bodies have different morphologic features: Coccoid,

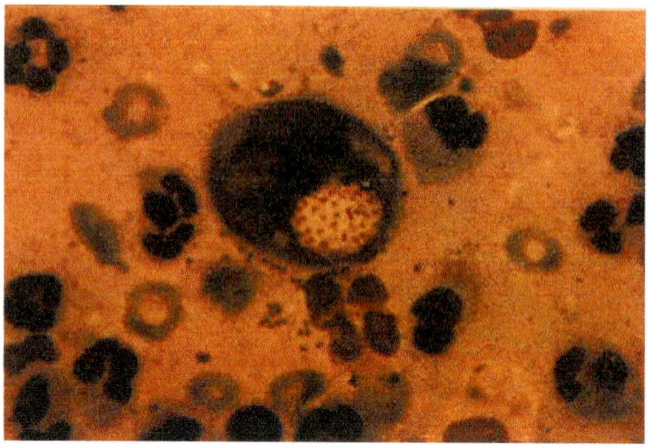

Fig. 15.5: Donovan bodies in large mononuclear cells

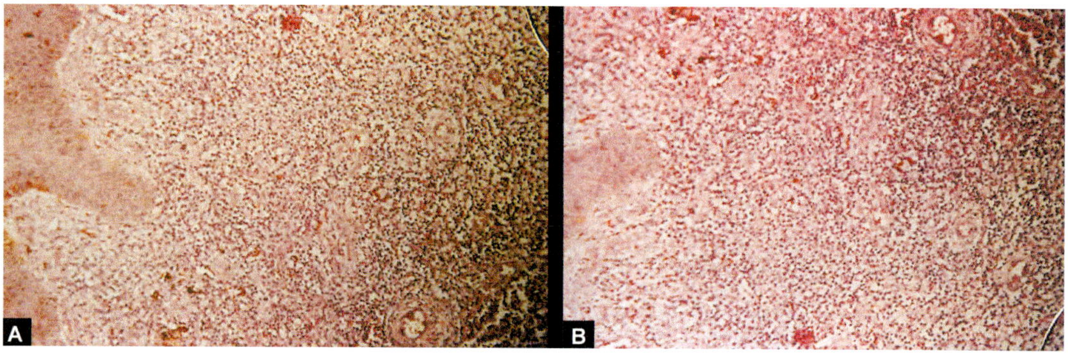

Figs 15.6A and B: Tissue section showing massive inflammatory infiltrate comprising plasma and mononuclear cells. Vascular dialatation showing endothelial proliferation (H and E x 400) *(Courtesy:* Sehgal et al. British Journal of Venereal Diseases 1984;60:45-7)

coccobacillary, or bacillary. Mature forms surrounded by a capsule are seen in some sections. They are easily identified in slow (over night) Giemsa-stained tissue sections (Appendix). The organisms in the tissue section are primarily intracytoplasmic clusters of coccobacillary forms taking a purplish to pink stain. They stand prominently over the background of faint blue cytoplasm surrounding the deep blue nuclei of the mononuclear cells. In addition, enlarged mono-nuclear cells with multiple cystic spaces containing Donovan bodies and eccentrically situated nuclei are uniformly conspicuous. They are difficult to identify in hematoxylin and eosin stained sections. Vascular changes (dilation, proliferation, or both) are predominant. Endothelial proliferation is a common feature, and proliferation of the tunica media may be seen.

The tissue sections show discontinuity in the epidermis, with ulcerations varying from mild to severe. Proliferation of the stratum spinosum (acanthosis) in the form of elongation of rete ridges is a constant feature of the hypertrophic variety. This, however, may also be seen in some of the ulcerative lesions. Similarly, pseudoepitheliomatous hyperplasia may also be a feature of the hypertrophic variant. Evidence of malignancy in the form of horn pearls, atypia of individual cells, or numerous mitotic figures is usually lacking. Neutrophilic sprinkling of both upper dermis and the epidermis is seen regularly; these occasionally form microabscesses (Fig. 15.8). The adnexae, fat, and muscle are conspicuously spared.

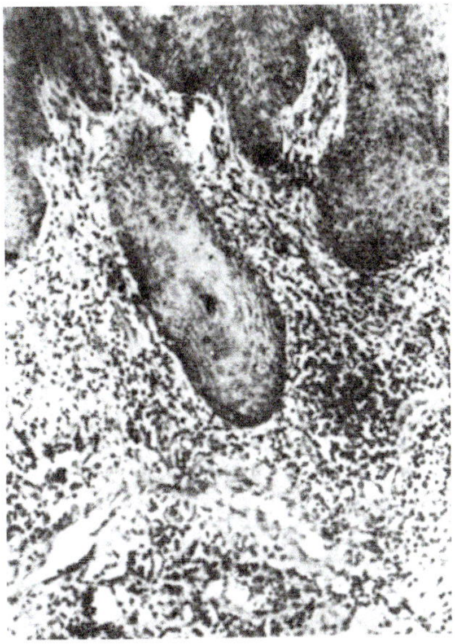

Fig. 15.7: Epidermal changes in the form of elongation of the rete ridges with intense inflammatory infiltrate primarily of mononuclear cells (H and E x 160) *(Courtesy:* Sehgal et al. British Journal of Venereal Disease 1984;60:45-7)

The possibility of donovanosis should be considered in all earnest in the differential diagnosis of genital ulcerations. At this juncture, it is worth while to recapitulate the other venereal and nonvenereal causes of genital ulcerations.

Chancroid

It is characterized by multiple, small, superficial, painful, dirty necrotic ulcers of varying sizes. The edges of the ulcers are undermined and surrounded by a narrow zone of erythema and edema. They are tender and bleed on touch. Inguinal bubo may be an accompaniment. Usually the bubo is a unilateral, unilocular, fluctuant, tender swelling with overlying taut and erythematous skin. The incubation period varies from 2 to 7 days. Dwarf chancroid is characterized by a small superficial ulcer. Giant chancroid is a large granulomatous ulcer as a consequence of a ruptured bubo extending to involve the surrounding skin. Follicular chancroids are seen in association with the hair follicles, while serpiginous chancroids are characterized by multiple ulcers coalescing to form a serpiginous pattern. Its phagedenic variant may cause extensive destruction of the genitals, associated with a foul smelling discharge. Demonstration of *Haemophilus ducreyi* in a Gram stained smear is diagnostic. Recovery of the organisms *in vitro* is, however, imperative for diagnosis.

Chancroidal Ulcers

These ulcers have recently been defined. They are single ulcers with the morphology of chancroid. Their incubation period is longer, 8 to 11 days, and they show an absence of lymphadenopathy. Modern culture techniques, which can be used to isolate *H. ducreyi* in a majority of chancroid cases, fail to demonstrate the organism from chancroidal ulcers. Instead, a polymicrobial flora may be isolated.

Herpes Progenitalis

Only rarely can this viral infection be mistaken for granuloma inguinale. It presents classically as grouped vesicular lesions on an erythematous base. The vesicles rupture in a day or two to form superficial, tender, polycyclic erosions on the genitalia. There may be a long history of recurrences and remissions. In early cases, scraping the floor of a vesicle gently with a scalpel, putting the material on a clean glass slide, and staining with Giemsa's stain reveals characteristic multinucleated giant cells in the smear. Cell culture technique is used to isolate the causative virus. The condition heals spontaneously.

Syphilis

Early syphilis comprises primary and secondary stages. The incubation period of the primary chancre varies from 10 to 90 days. It is a painless, erythematous, indurated papule that erodes to form an ulcer. The ulcer is painless, clean, well-defined, and indurated and has a raw exuding surface. It resembles a button glued to the skin or the mucous membrane. The secondary stage is recognized by an asymptomatic polymorphic bilateral and symmetrical rash, mucous patches, snail track ulcers, and generalized lymphadenopathy with the classic features just listed. Distinct clinical variants comprising syphilids of various morphology, namely macular, papular, pustular, follicular, annular, psoriasiform and condylomata lata may be found. The condylomata, in particular, are quite frequent and are evident as flat-topped, greyish-white eruptions with oozing of serum, primarily on the genitals, anus, and axillae. Demonstration of *Treponema pallidum* from the secondary lesions is confirmatory.

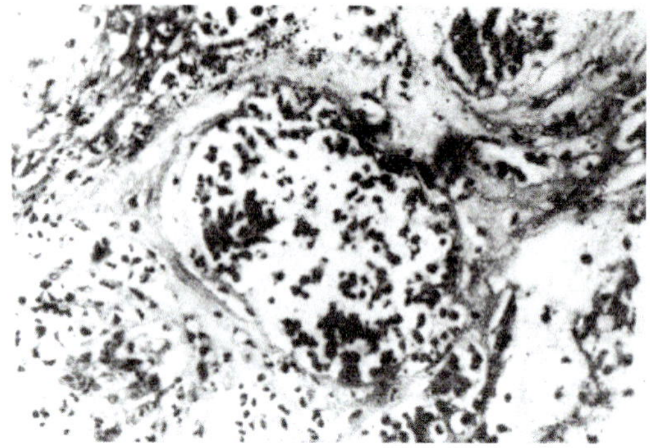

Fig. 15.8: Ulcer with microabscess formation (H and E × 400) (*Courtesy:* Sehgal et al. British Journal of Venereal Diseases, 1984:60:45-47)

Tertiary syphilis is rarely seen nowadays. The ulcerative variety has a punched-out appearance with sharp vertical edges and a dull-gray, chamois like slough base. The nodular and psoriasiform type are unlikely to be mistaken for granuloma inguinale.

Lymphogranuloma Venereum (LGV)

Granuloma inguinale and LGV are morphologically distinct from each other; however, the earlier nomenclature (granuloma venereum vs lymphogranuloma venereum) may be a cause of confusion. LGV presents initially as transient, herpetiform vesicular lesions on the genitalia. These heal within a week. After 2 to 8 weeks, the patient has inguinal lymphadenitis and constitutional manifestations. The adenitis is multilocular, tender, and nonfluctuant. The overlying skin is usually normal unless suppuration occurs, in which case multiple discharging sinuses are formed. Lymph nodes above and below the inguinal ligament are involved (groove sign), with the inguinal ligament appearing as a groove between the two lymph node masses. A positive intradermal Frei's test and the modern serologic techniques of complement fixation and microimmunoassay further differentiate LGV from granuloma inguinale. *Chlamydia trachomatis,* the causative organism, may also be cultured from material taken from a bubo or from the genital. The late manifestations of LGV due to lymphatic obstruction may be very similar to those seen in granuloma inguinale-induced pseudoelephantiasis. Elephantiasis, leading to enormous hypertrophy of the genitalia, is the usual feature in such cases.

Candidosis

This common condition is due to *Candida albicans,* an opportunistic yeast. It presents in men as balanoposthitis with fissuring of the prepuce. A moist, sodden, whitish plaque is seen. Its removal reveals an erythematous erosive area. There may be isolated, peripheral vesiculopustules. Demonstration of the fungus is simple. A surface scraping of the lesions mounted in 10 percent potassium hydroxide solution shows budding pseudohyphae in abundance. There is frequently concomitant diabetes mellitus.

Traumatic Ulcers

These are seen in men in the form of sharply demarcated, usually linear cuts on the genitalia. The history is that the condition developed or was noticed immediately after sexual intercourse. The tendency is spontaneous healing, if further intercourse is avoided. However, if a sexually transmitted condition is superimposed, the lesion changes its morphologic characteristics.

Squamous Cell Carcinoma

Squamous cell carcinoma of the penis may pose a diagnostic problem. The resemblance to granuloma inguinale can be close, both conditions exhibiting a granulomatous, ulcerated growth with hypertrophic rolled-over edges. In later stages, of course, involvement of the inguinal lymph nodes occurs in carcinoma. These are firm to hard and subsequently become fixed to deeper structures. In the earlier stages, both a tissue smear and a biopsy are prerequisites. Histopathologically, although epidermal changes can be similar, the presence of numerous mitoses, irregularity, bizarre patterns of nuclei, and horn pearls in carcinoma help differentiate the two conditions.

Skin Tuberculosis

Scrofuloderma may present in the inguinal region as discharging sinuses and ulcers. Usually, however, the underlying lymph nodes can be felt as a matted mass to which the sinuses are fixed. They are necrotic and friable, have undermined edges, and have a bluish margin. Tuberculosis verrucosa cutis may, very rarely, present in the genitoinguinal region. In such cases, confusion with the hypertrophic variant of granuloma inguinale may arise. Histopathology provides the answer: skin tuberculosis shows areas of caseation necrosis with a surrounding granuloma of epithelioid cells and lymphocytes. An admixture of polymorphonuclear cells may be present. Special staining with Ziehl-Neelsen stain will reveal acid-fast bacilli.

Filariasis

The late stage of filaria presents as elephantiasis of the genitalia. However, the absence of genital ulcerations in the past, an initial acute episode of fever with (usually) scrotal swelling, and microfilaria seen on a peripheral blood smear taken at night, all distinguish it from granuloma inguinale.

Fixed Drug Eruption

This can be diagnosed by its salient morphologic features, namely, single, well-defined, superficial, erosive lesions with no regional lymphadenopathy. The lesion is preceded or accompanied by itching and burning. Patients often do not relate their complaints to the use of drugs. Drug eruption is especially important in developing countries. A drug history should, therefore, be pursued thoroughly and systematically. In cases where the nature of the drug is not known to the patient, eliciting the complaint for which the drug was taken may be helpful. Provoking the lesion(s) with the suspecting drug confirms the diagnosis and may help prevent recurrences in the future. It also allays the patient's anxiety regarding the venereal origin of the signs.

TREATMENT

Granuloma inguinale has long presented difficulties in treatment. Until the early part of this century, surgery was employed to excise the lesion, along with the margin of normal tissue. The resulting scar often broke down to cause a recurrence. Earlier, potassium antimony tartrate was used in a 1 to 2 percent solution in normal saline or in 5 percent dextrose and given intravenously, repeated on alternate days. Although this was successful for disease in the early stages, chronic cases were very resistant. Fouadin, a trivalent antimony preparation, was also used, as were other antimonials. The toxicity and antimony fastness (recurrent lesions developing resistance) were the main drawbacks of antimonial therapy.

Drugs

Streptomycin

Barton *et al* first used this drug in the treatment of granuloma inguinale. Greenblatt *et al* organized the first large-scale trial of streptomycin and attempted to rationalize the dosage schedule. A dosage of 4 g per day in divided doses for 5 days was found to be optimal. Donovan bodies disappeared from the lesions an average of 6 days after initiation of therapy, while healing occurred 1 to 2 weeks after cessation of treatment. There were a few relapses. In another well-documented study. Kupperman *et al* found that streptomycin in total dose of more than 20 g resulted in cure in all cases, while recurrences were experienced with smaller dosages. Rajam and Rangiah, however, had commendable results with smaller (1-2 g) daily doses over a period of 10 days; however, failure of streptomycin later was reported from India and abroad. The high risk of side effects has further discouraged its use.

Tetracyclines

Oxytetracycline was found to be effective in optimal doses of 2 g per day by mouth over a period of 10 to 14 days. Chlortetracycline was found to be equally effective, the optimal dosage being the same as that for oxytetracycline. Low cost, high efficacy and ease of administration make tetracyclines the drug of first choice in granuloma inguinale.

Cotrimoxazole

Although sulfonamides are ineffective in the treatment of granuloma inguinale, a combination of sulfamethoxazole and trimethoprim has been found useful. In a subsequent follow-up, only 2 of 116 patients had recurrence after administration of two tablets twice a day for 10 to 15 days. This was confirmed by Rosen *et al* Subramanian, and Spagnole *et al.* The treatment schedule is given in Table 15.2.

In addition, recent World Health Organization (WHO) guidelines for the treatment of granuloma inguinale are included in Table 15.3 to exercise judicious option.

Table 15.2: Treatment schedule for granuloma inguinale

Drugs	*Daily dosage*	*Total doses*	*Durations*
1. Tetracyclines (oral)			
i. Terramycin	2 g in four equal divided doses	20-40 g	10-20 days
ii. Aureomycin	2 g in four equal divided doses	—do—	—do—
2. Streptomycin (intramuscular)	2 g in two equal doses	20-40 g	10-20 days
3. Cotrimoxazole (oral) (trimethoprim, 80 mg plus sulfamethoxazole, 400 mg)	2 tablets two times a day	40-60 tablets	10-15 days

Note: Treatment may be prolonged if recovery is partial/incomplete.

Table 15.3 : Granuloma inguinale treatment: WHO guidelines

Treatment should be continued until all lesions have epithelialized
Recommended regimen
Azithromycin 1 gm on the first day and then 500mg every day
Or Doxycycline 100 mg orally twice a day
Alternative regimens
Erythromycin 500 mg, orally 4 times a day
Or Tetracycline 500 mg, orally 4 times a day
Or Trimethoprim 80 mg with sulphamethoxazole 400 mg, orally 2 tablets twice daily for a minimum of 14 days

Note: The addition of a parentral aminoglycoside such as gentamicin should be considered in HIV positive patients. Appropriate surgical intervention may be needed in pseudoelephantiasis and other complications.

FURTHER READING

1. Greenblatt RB. Management of chancroid, granuloma inguinale, lymphogranuloma venereum in general practice. US public Health Service Publication No 255,1953.
2. Miller P. Donovanosis: Control or eradication? A situation review of aboriginal and Torres strait islander populations in Australia. Canberra, Health and Aged Care 2001;1-37.
3. O'Farrell N. Donovanosis: an update. Int J STD AIDS 2001; 12: 423-7.
4. Rajam V, Rangiah PN. Donovanosis. World Health Organisation Monograph Series No 20, 1954.
5. Sehgal VN, Prasad AL. The clinical profile of donovanosis is non-endemic area. Dermatologica 1984;168:273-8.
6. Sehgal VN, Prasad AL. Donovanosis: current concepts. Int J Dermatol 1986;25:8-16.
7. Sehgal VN, Jain MK. Pattern of epidemics of donovanosis in the 'non-endemic' region. Int J Dermatol 1986;27:396-9.
8. Sehgal VN, Jain MK, Sharma VK. Pseudoelephantiasis induced by donovanosis. Genitourin Med 1987;63: 54-6.
9. Sehgal VN. Donovanosis (Granuloma Inguinale) (1st edn): Jaypee Brothers Medical Publisher, New Delhi, 1988.

Chapter 16

Genital Herpes Infection

INTRODUCTION

Genital herpes infections is caused by herpes simplex virus type-1 and type-2 (HSV-1 and 2). It contains a double stranded linear DNA, a surrounding icosahedral protein capsid consisting of 162 capsomers, a tegument composed of fibrillar material (protein), and an impermeable envelop, consisting of lipids, polyamines, and virus specific glycoproteins. The two different serotypes (1 and 2) of HSV can be differentiated by serologic, biologic (tissue culture plaque and neurotropic differentiation), and biochemical (DNA homology) studies.

Humans are the only natural host of HSV. The virus is first introduced into a susceptible host by direct mucocutaneous contact with infectious material. The viral envelop fuses with the plasma membrane. The capsid is uncoated in the cytoplasm, and the core DNA enters the nucleus. Early transcription follows, utilizing the host DNA dependent RNA polymerase. The necessary virus coded enzymes are synthesized and viral DNA replication occurs. The new herpes virus is assembled in the nucleus, and the envelopment takes place at the inner lamella of the nuclear membranes. Subsequently, the virus emerges from the infected cell.

After epithelial inoculation, the virus travels along the sensory nerves to reach the regional sensory ganglia, via retrograde intraxonal transport. This process starts 24 hours after epithelial inoculation. In the ganglia, the virus is dormant. It may be reactivated either by ganglionic or skin trigger. In the former, on reactivation the virus travels down the peripheral nerve to the epidermal cells, producing skin lesions. In the latter, microfoci of infection are continuously produced but are eliminated by the immune defences. However, if the immunity is lowered, these microfoci become symptomatic. Reactivation may be triggered by fever, systemic infection, menses, physical trauma, emotional stress, sunburn, and administration of corticosteroids and immunosuppressive drugs.

CLINICAL FEATURES

It may manifest either as primary or recurrent infection. The primary infection indicates an individual's first exposure to either HSV-1 or HSV-2. This may result in the production of neutralizing antibodies, cytotoxic antibodies, and complement fixation antibodies. The incubation period for primary infection is 3 to 12 days. It runs a clinical course of 1 to 3 weeks. The lesions are usually extensive and accompanied by constitutional symptoms of headache, fever, and malaise. Virus excretion may persist for 15 to 42 days. After primary infection, HSV remains dormant in sensory ganglia and may be periodically reactivated to cause recurrent episodes. The recurrent lesions are much less severe, restricted to smaller areas and constitutional symptoms are mild or absent. The lesions may heal in

7 to 10 days. The primary infection may also be asymptomatic. There is only serologic evidence of subclinical primary infection. In such patients, the first clinical manifestation of herpes is known as first episode infection.

Primary Infection

It begins with a prodrome of severe localized tenderness and accompanying fever and constitutional symptoms. There is then an eruption of grouped vesicles on erythematous base. The regional lymph nodes are enlarged and tender. Purulent, malodorous discharge may accompany oral or vulvovaginal infection. Urethritis may be accompanied by dysuria and/or discharge. Tenesmus and constipation may be associated with anorectal infection.

Herpetic Gingivostomatitis

It is heralded by high fever, and malaise. The grouped vesicle on erythematous base appear in oral cavity. They may break to form polycyclic erosions and ulcers. They affect the oral mucosa, tongue, and tonsils. Regional lymph node may be enlarged and tender. Tonsillitis and/or pharyngitis may be present. The patient usually has pain, foul breath, difficulty in opening the mouth, and swallowing. This may produce dehydration and acidosis. The herpetic gingivostomatitis needs to be differentiated from streptococcal infection, infectious mononucleosis, thrush, erythema-multiforme, Stevens-Johnson syndrome, Behçet's syndrome, pemphigus vulgaris, and herpangina.

Inoculation Herpes

It develops on the paronychial region. The virus is inoculated as a result of trauma. There is appearance of grouped vesicles over an erythematous base, the 'herpetic whit-low'. Regional lymph nodes are enlarged and tender.

Herpetic Vulvovaginitis

It is heralded by marked erythema and edema of the vulva. The grouped vesicle appear over erythematous base. The vesicles rupture within 24 to 48 hours after eruption to form polycyclic erosions. Constitutional symptoms of fever, headache, and malaise precede and accompany herpetic vulvovaginitis. Regional lymph nodes the enlarged and tender. There may be vaginal discharge. Urinary retention may be a complication. The lesions usually heal within 2 to 6 weeks.

Herpetic Cervicitis

It is often asymptomatic. However, it is a risk to the fetus in a pregnant woman. Herpes virus contracted *in utero* may result in anomalies in the newborn like microcephaly, microphthalmos, encephalitis, chorioretinitis, and intracerebral calcification. Maternal genital herpetic infection may also be associated with abortions, stillbirths, and premature delivery. Seventy percent of neonatal herpes simplex are caused by HSV-2 and acquired as the child passes through the infected birth canal. The neonatal infection may be localized skin infection or systemic and present as encephalitis, hepatitis, pneumonia, and coagulopathy. The risk of infection to the neonate is 3 to 5 percent in recurrent infection and 50 percent in case of primary infection. Herpetic infection during labor necessitates caesarian section before the membranes rupture or within four hours of it.

Primary Herpes Genitalis in Men

It starts with pain, burning, and redness over the genitalia. This is followed by the eruption of grouped vesicles, which rupture to form erosions (Fig. 16.1). The lesions are localized to the glans penis and pubic region. Inguinal lymph nodes are enlarged and tender. Constitutional symptoms are usually present. Urethral discharge may be an accompaniment.

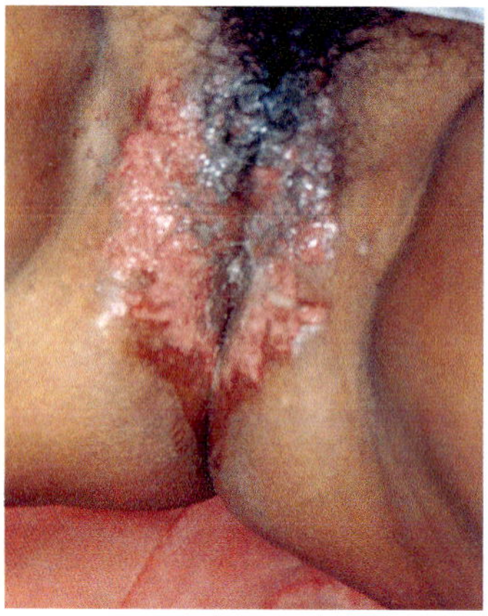

Fig. 16.1: Herpes progenitalis

Anorectal Herpes

It is characterized by the typical vesicular eruption which subsequently ulcerates. Tenesmus and constipation may accompany anorectal herpes.

Disseminated Herpes Simplex

This may be encountered in infants and children up to 3 years of age.

Malnourishment, kwashiorkor, measles, immunosuppressive drugs, and atopic dermatitis, predispose to disseminated infection. It may also develop in patients with acquired immunodeficiency syndrome (AIDS). The disease begins with gingivostomatitis and then disseminates to involve the liver, gastrointestinal tract, and central nervous system. Viremia may result in death.

Recurrent Infection

There is a prodrome of mild tenderness, and slight erythematous blush followed by the eruption of grouped vesicles. The vesicles, initially clear turn purulent and then dry to form crust. Healing occurs within 7 to 10 days. Tender regional lymphadenopathy accompanies recurrent herpes. The following complications may develop:

- Herpetic pharyngitis
- Herpetic urethritis
- Aseptic meningitis
- Urinary retention
- Tenesmus and constipation
- Erythema multiforme and Stevens-Johnson syndrome
- Dissemination of herpetic infection in immunosuppressed individuals
- Prenatal and neonatal herpes simplex infections
- Women with recurrent herpes progenitalis are prone to cervical carcinoma and advised yearly Papanicolaou smears.

DIAGNOSIS

The diagnosis of herpes simplex is clinical. It may be supplemented by various diagnostic procedures:

- Cytologic smear of the vesicle reveals large multinucleate giant cells containing 8 to 10 nuclei, varying in shape and size. An intranuclear inclusion body may be identified (Figs 16.2A and B).
- *Skin biopsy reveals:* (1) an intraepidermal lesion in mid to upper epidermis, (2) ballooning and/or reticular degeneration of cells, (3) acantholytic cells, (4) large, multinucleated viral giant cells
- Virus may be cultured from the vesicle fluid
- Direct immunofluorescence using monoclonal antibody
- Identification of the virus under electron microscope.

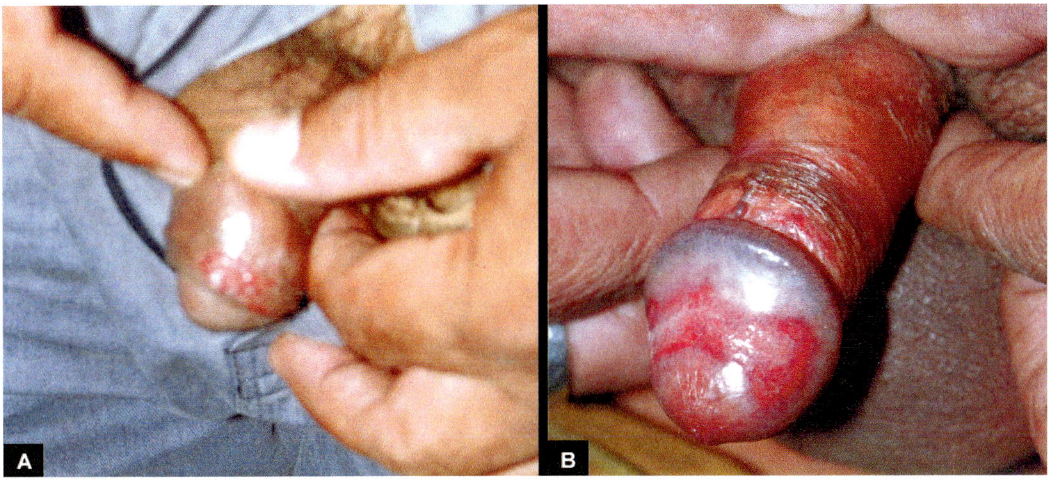

Figs 16.2A and B: Tzanck smear. Multinucleate giant cells

TREATMENT

The treatment of herpes simplex may be considered into symptomatic and specific. The antiherpetic drugs are classified as:

- *First generation:* (1) Idoxuridine, (2) Trifluridine, (3) Adenine arabinoside.
- *Second generation:* (1) Acyclovir, (2) Bromovinyldeoxyuridine (BVdU), (3) Fluoroiodoara-cytosine (FIAC), (4) Phosphonoformate (PFA)
- *Third generation:* (1) Adenosine arabinoside 5'-monophosphate, (2) Acyclovir analogue namely dihydroxypropoxy-methyl-guanine (DHPG).
- *Others:* (1) Interferon, (2) Ribavarin, (3) Isoprinosine

Acyclovir is most widely used antiviral agent. It is an acyclic nucleoside analogue, with activity against herpes simplex (HSV-1 and 2) and herpes zoster virus. It is as elective substrate for the viral thymidine kinase. The virus specific thymidine kinase concentrates acyclovir in the herpes infected cells by phosphorylating 'it to monophosphate derivative. Cellular kinase then converts the monophosphate derivative to acyclovir triphosphate. This is a competitive inhibitor of viral DNA polymerase and DNA chain terminated or land inhibits viral DNA synthesis. It reduces viral shedding, decreases the time for healing and crusting, and reduces pain. It also prolongs remission, however, recurrence occurs on stopping the drug. The effect of oral acyclovir on recurrent herpes is as impressive as on primary infection, provided the treatment is begun within 48 hours of the onset of signs and symptoms. Intravenous acyclovir is used for the management of potentially catastrophic herpes infections. Topical acyclovir has a modest effect on primary and first episode of herpes progenitalis if begun within 72 hours, however, it does not abort recurrent infections. The schedule of treatment are outline in Table 16.1.

Although, the afore mentioned treatment may still be valid in remote regions of developing countries yet taking stock of recent World Health Organization (WHO) guidelines is in order and should be given due cognizance (Table 16.2).

Table 16.1: Genital herpes infection treatment

Type of infection	*Specific treatment*	*Symptomatic treatment*
1. Primary and first episode herpes infection	a. 200 mg of acyclovir 5 times a day for 5 days. Begin treatment within 72 hours of the onset of signs and symptoms. b. Topical application of 5 percent acyclovir ointment (Herperax) every 3 hours	1. Cool compresses with Burrow's solution for for 10 min, 3 to 4 times a day. 2. Cleansing mouthwashes with tetracycline suspension or potassium permanganate in herpetic gingivostomatitis
2. Recurrent herpes	800 mg of acyclovir twice a day or 200 mg five times a day for 5 days Begin treatment within 48 hours of the onset of signs	3. Sitz's bath for Vulvo vaginitis and anorectal herpes. 4. Salicylates and other non-steroidal anti-inflammatory drugs and symptoms 5. Topical antibiotics to cure secondary infection

Table 16.2: Genital herpes infection treatment: WHO guidelines

Recommended regimens

First episode herpes

Acyclovir 200 mg, 5 times a day for 7 days.

Or

Acyclovir 400 mg, 3 times a day for 7 days

Or

Valacyclovir 1 gm orally twice a day for 7 days

Or

Fanciclovir 250 mg orally three times a day for 7 days

Recommended regimen for recurrent infection

Acyclovir 200 mg, orally 5 times a day

Or

Acyclovir 500 mg mg orally 3 times a day for 5 days

Or

Acyclovir 800 mg orally twice a day for 5 days

Or

Valacyclovir 500 mg bd, for 5 days

Or

Valacyclovir 1000 mg orally once daily for 5 days

Or

Famciclovir 125 mg orally twice a day for 5 days

Recommended regimens for suppressive therapy

Acyclovir 400 mg twice daily continuously

Or

Valacyclovir 500 mg orally once daily

Or

Valacyclovir 1000 mg orally once daily

Or

Famciclovir 250 mg orally twice daily

Note: Some experts recommend discontinuing acyclovir after one year of continuous use so that the recurrence rate can be reassessed. The lowest continuous dose that will suppress recurrences in an individual can be determined empirically.

Recommended regimen for severe disease

Acyclovir 5-10 mg/kg IV, 8 hourly for 5-7 days or until clinical resolution is attained

Recommended regimen for severe herpes simplex lesions with coinfection with HIV

Acyclovir 400 mg, 3-5 times a daily, until clinical resolution is attained

Recommended regimen for neonates

Acyclovir 10 mg/kg intravenously, 3 times a day for 10-21 days

FURTHER READING

1. Corey L. First episode, recurrent, and asymptomatic herpes simplex infection. J Am Acad Dermatol 1988; 18: 169-72.
2. Cusini M, Ghislanzoni M. The importance of diagnosing genital herpes. J Antimicrob Chemother 2001; 47: 9-16.
3. Flowers FP, Araujo OE, Turner LA. Recent advances in antiherpetic drugs. Int J Dermatol 1988; 27:612-6.
4. Goldman BD. Herpes serology for dermatologists. Arch Dermatol 2000;136:1158-61.
5. Landy HJ, Grossman JH. Herpes simplex virus. Obstet Gynecol Clin North Am 1989;16:495-515.
6. Leung DT, Sacks SI. Current recommendations for the treatment of genital herpes. Drugs 2000;60:1329-52.
7. Marques AR, Straus SE. Herpes simplex type 2 infections—an update. Dis Mon 2000; 46: 325-59.
8. Olmscheid B, Boyle BA. Behavioral interventions and host mucosal factors in transmission of HIV. AIDS Read 2001;11:238-9.
9. O'Farrell N. Increasing prevalence of genital herpes in developing countries: implications for heterosexual HIV transmission and STI control programmes. Sex Transm Infect 1999;75:377-84.
10. Sandhaus S. Genital herpes in pregnant and non-pregnant women. Nurse Pract 2001;26:15-6.
11. Thomas DJ. Sexually transmitted viral infections: epidemiology and treatment. J Obstet Gynecol Neonatal Nurs 2001;30:316-23.
12. Tetrault I, Boivin G. Recent advances in management of genital herpes. Can Fam Physician 2000;46: 1622-9.
13. Tariq A, Ross JD. Viral sexually transmitted infections: current management strategies. J Clin Pharm Ther 1999; 24:409-14.

Chapter 17

Minor Sexually Transmitted Diseases

INTRODUCTION

Some infections of the genital tract such as trichomoniasis, candidosis, scabies and pediculosis are included under this group, for they may be transmitted sexually, although not exclusively. The salient features of these diseases form the subject of the text.

TRICHOMONIASIS

Trichomoniasis is an infection of the genital tract by *Trichomonas vaginalis.*

Epidemiology

Trichomoniasis occurs all over the world. It infects both sexes, in the third and the fourth decades. It is usually transmitted through coitus, but female to female transmission may also occur in poor sanitary contexts.

Etiology

Trichomonas vaginalis is its causative organism. It is an oval or pear-shaped organism of the size of 10-30 μ. It has an oval nucleus, from its posterior end an elongation termed axostyle is seen. In front of the nucleus there are small rounded structures-blepharoplast from which five flagella arise. One of these flagella gets attached to the undulating membrane posteriorly. The free flagella with the undulating membrane make the characteristic movements (Fig. 17.1).

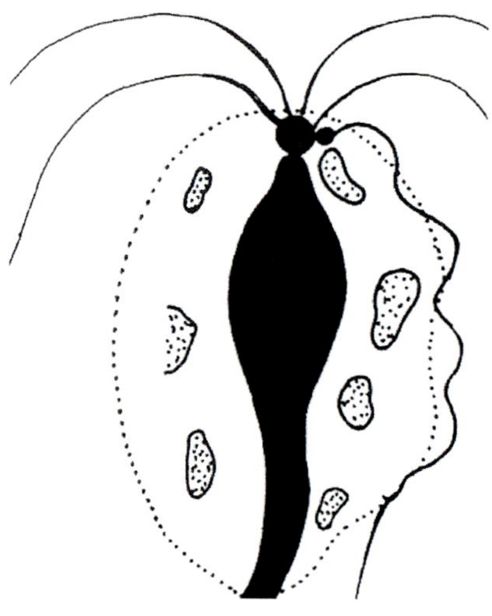

Fig. 17.1: *Trichomonas vaginalis*

Incubation Period

It varies from four days to three weeks.

Clinical Features

Usually, it is a silent condition. In females, it may manifest as vaginitis, vulvitis and urethritis. The patient may report with leukorrhea, dyspareunia and irritation of the genitals. The examination may reveal erythematous, edematous vaginal wall with copious, frothy, foul-smelling exudate. Similarly, vulvitis and urethritis may be noticed. It may have concomitant gonococcal infection. In males, the condition is usually asymptomatic or may manifest as mild urethritis, characterized by burning micturition and scanty mucoid or mucopurulent discharge. It may also cause balanitis.

Diagnosis

The demonstration of the organism in the secretions, centrifugate or urine, or vaginal or urethral scrapings, by direct wet smear or culture, is diagnostic. Nevertheless, it is imperative to investigate for other concomitant venereal infections like gonorrhea and candidosis.

Treatment

Spontaneous cure may be contemplated in some cases. Metronidazole (Flagyl) is the drug of choice. It is recommended in the dosage of 600 mg per day in three equal divided doses, for a period of seven days, up to a total dose of 4.2 gm. The symptoms and signs may disappear with this treatment. It may also be administered in a single dose regime of 2 gm. Infection resistant "to metronidazole has also been found.

Tinidazole

Tinidazole (Tiniba) is an established, highly effective, orally active, anti-protozoal drug. It is the latest synthetic imidazole derivative for the oral treatment of trichomoniasis. It is either given as 300 mg daily for 7 days or 2 gm straight, as a single dose. Simultaneous treatment of male/female partner is imperative.

CANDIDIASIS OF THE GENITAL TRACT

Candidiasis is a *Candida* infection of the genital tract characterized by irritation and discharge.

Epidemiology

Candida albicans responsible for candidosis is commensal in the genitals in health, but may turn pathogenic under favorable conditions like pregnancy, malnutrition, diabetes and on treatment with wide-spectrum antibiotics, immunosuppressive drugs and oral contraceptives. It may affect males and females of any age group. Hot humid climate and unhygienic conditions may favor the infection.

Etiology

Candidiasis is caused by *Candida albicans.* It is identified by the spores and pseudomycelia in 10 percent KOH preparations. The organism grows readily on Sabouraud's medium. It may be transmitted by the sexual intercourse.

Clinical Features

It is usually transmitted through sexual contact. Nearly 50 percent of male contacts of women with candidal infection, harbour *C. albicans.* The male patient usually complains of intense itching, burning or irritation over the perputial orifice. The prepuce may be difficult to retract and fissured. There is a scant whitish subpreputial discharge. If retraction is possible, the inner surface of the prepuce and glans penis are found to be inflamed. They are erythematous and studded at places with white patches (Figs 17.2A and B). Erosions may also be present. Itchy and scaly lesions may be present over the penile shaft and scrotum and may extend to involve the groins also.

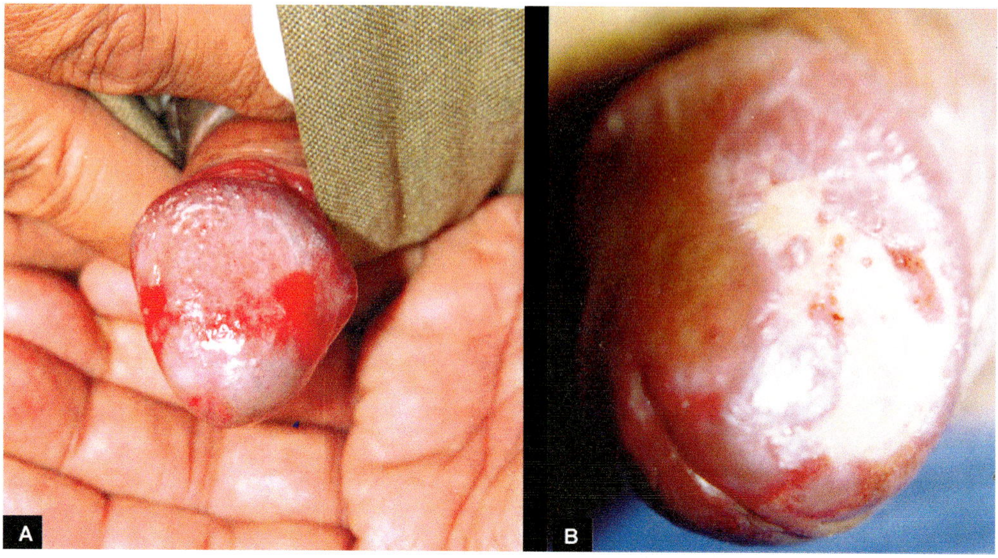

Figs 17.2A and B: Candidosis glans

Candidiasis of the genital tract may be asymptomatic in females. Some may complain of intense vulval and/or vaginal irritation with or without vaginal discharge. The latter is characteristically white and thick. There may be history of dyspareunia and/or dysuria. Examination of the vulva reveals erythematous and edematous mucosae studded with white curdy patches. Fissures and erosions may be present. Perspeculum examination of the vagina reveals a similar picture on the vaginal mucosa with 'cheese'-like secretions covering the vaginal portion of the cervix. The white vaginal plaques are difficult to remove and leave bleeding points. The vaginal discharge may be watery and its pH is below 5.

DIAGNOSIS

The clinical suspicion of candidiasis may be confirmed by smear examination and/or culture.

Candida albicans is a dimorphic fungus with both yeast and mycelial forms.

- Skin scrapings or other specimens are examined microscopically for budding yeast, pseudohypae or hypae after the addition of 10 percent KOH solution to the slide preparation. As *Candida* may be seen on normal skin or mucosae as well, only their abundant presence is significant. Demonstration of mycelial form indicates colonization and tissue invasion and is, therefore, of greater significance.
- Cultures can be obtained readily on Sabouraud's and ordinary bacteriological culture media. Colonies are creamy white, smooth, and have a distinct yeasty odor.
- A rapid method of identifying *C. albicans* is based on its ability to form germ tubes within two hours when incubated in human serum at 37°C (Reynold-Braude phenomenon).

Treatment

Largely candidiasis is treated by topical application of one to two percent aqueous solution of gentian violet, nystatin cream (Mycostatin) or by inserting nystatin vaginal tablets (Mycostatin vaginal) for a period of two weeks or more. Trichomycin, another polyene derivative, is useful for it is not only effective against candidiasis, but also against trichomoniasis. In case the precipitating cause(s) are

Table 17.1: Treatment of candidiasis

Clinical form	*Treatment*
1. Vulvovaginal candidiasis	Anticandidal prepration, as pessaries or cream inserted intravaginally. In addition, topical anticandidals may be applied over the vulva, Male partner may need simultaneous treatment. 1. Clotrimazole 100 mg vaginal tablet (I midil, Surfaz or Canesten vaginal tablet). Insert one tablet high in the vagina, at bedtime, for 6 consecutive nights or 2. Miconazole nitrate 200 mg vaginal pessary (Gynodaktrin ovule). Insert one tablet in vagina, for 3 consecutive nights or 3. Econazole nitrate 150 mg (Econazole vaginal). Insert one tablet in vagina, for 3 consecutive nights. or 4. Nystatin 100,000 units vaginal tablet (Mycostatin vaginal), 1 to 2 tablets may be inserted in the vagina for 2 weeks 5. Miconazole nitrate 2 percent W/W gel (Gynodaktrin) applied intravaginally at bedtime, for 7 to 14 days or 6. Ciclopirox olamine 10 mg per g cream (Laprox vaginal cream), 5 mg inserted in the vagina at bedtime with applicator for 12 to 14 days OR **Recalcitrant cases may require** 1. One tablet Nystatin (500,000 Units), four times a day for 2 weeks or 2. 200 mg of ketoconazole, twice a day for 5 days.
2. Candidal balanoposthitis	Topical anticandidal preparations, applied twice a day for 10 to 14 days. 1. Clotrimazole 1 percent cream (Canesten, I mid II) 2. Micronazole nitrate 2 percent (Micogel, Daktarin) 3. Ciclopirox olamine 10 mg per g (Laprox) **Recalcitrant cases may require** 1. One tablet Nystatin (500, 000 units), four times a day or 2. 200 mg of ketoconazole, twice a day for 5 days

known they should be accordingly eliminated or treated. The latter is absolutely essential for achieving quick therapeutic response. The details are outlined in Table 17.1.

SCABIES

Scabies is a contagious parasitic disease characterized by generalized nocturnal itching with a typical rash distributed on the body folds.

Epidemiology

It is seen all over the world with its recent resurgence in some countries. It is transmitted from one infected individual to another directly or through fomites. It may be transmitted through sexual contact. Overcrowding, unhygienic conditions and cold climate may predispose the individual to the disease.

Etiology

It is caused by *Sarcoptes scabiei var hominis* which can be isolated from the burrows of scabies. The male mite dies after copulation, while the female lays 20-25 eggs, which hatch in about three days.

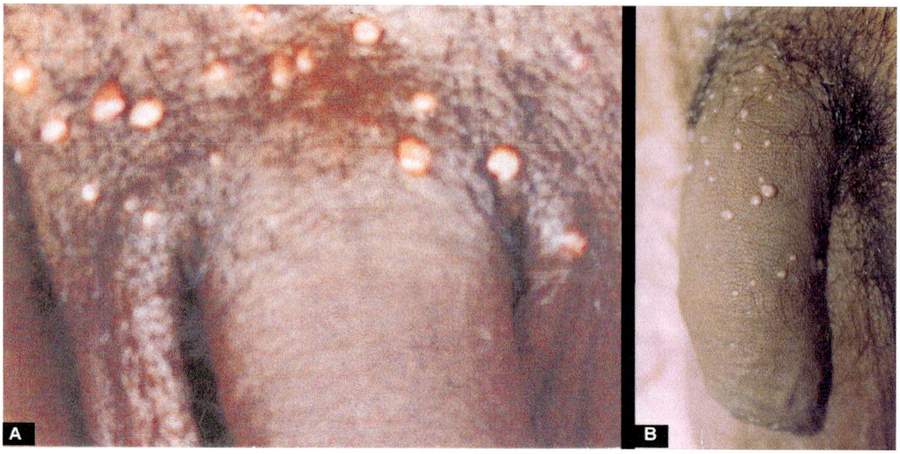

Figs 17.3A and B: Scabies shaft of the penis

The parasite reaches the adult stage in 7-14 days, thus completing the cycle.

Incubation Period

It varies from two to six weeks.

Clinical Features

The nocturnal itching is invariably the hallmark of the disease. The typical lesions are burrows, papules, vesicles, pustules and crusted lesions. They are characteristically distributed on the genitals (Figs 17.3A to C) and medial side of the thighs, in addition to the interdigital spaces, the elbow joints, the anterior axillary folds and the umbilicus.

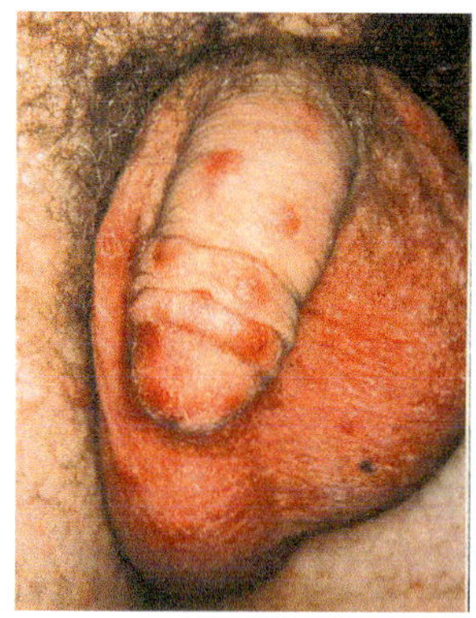

Fig. 17.3C: Scabies

Diagnosis

It is almost certain in the presence of positive family history, itching at night, and the distribution of the lesions on the scabetic sites. The diagnosis may be confirmed by demonstrating the parasite from the burrows.

Treatment

It consists of local application of either 25 percent benzyl benzoate (Ascabiol), ten percent sulphur ointment, 0.1 percent gamma benzene hexachloride (Lorexane) in lotion or cream or 6 percent of monosulfiram (Tetmosol) solution in methylated spirit. Two or three consecutive applications of either of the medicaments after an initial thorough scrub bath are adequate. Their contacts should also be simultaneously treated (Table 17.2).

PEDICULOSIS PUBIS

Pediculosis pubis is a parasitic infestation of the groins, characterized by pruritus and skin eruptions.

Table 17.2: Scabies treatment

Scabicidal agent	*Mode of application*	*Number of applications*	*Other measures*
1. 25% Benzyl benzoate for adults 12.5% for children (Ascabiol)	Apply to the whole of skin surface below the neck after a hot scrub bath	3 applications at 12 hours intervals followed by a bath	Clothes, bed clothes may be laundered. New washed set of clothes should be worn after treatment
2. 1% Gamma benzene hexachloride (Gab, Scarab)	—do—	Single application. Bath after 24 hours.	—do— Avoid application on face and in children as it is an irritant
3. 0.5% Malathion solution	—do—	—do—	—do—
4. 10% Crotamiton	May be applied on whole of the body	Two applications at 12 hours interval, followed by a bath	Usually preferred in infants and small children
5. 10% precipitate sulphur in petrolatum	Rarely used	—	Irritant and it stains the clothes
6. Monosulfiram (Tetmesol soap)	To be used as soap prior to applying other scabicidal agents	— —	
7. Topical Thiabendazole	—	—	—

Epidemiology

It is seen all over the world. It is common in unhygienic persons with poor socioeconomic status. It occurs both in males and females.

Etiology

It is caused by crab louse-*Phthirus pubis*-transmitted usually by sexual contacts. The pubic hair is their main habitat, but they are often found on the hair of the abdomen and the thighs.

Clinical Features

Intense itching is the cardinal clinical symptom. The disease is characterized by excoriation, secondary infection and blood crusts. In addition tiny pigmented macules, may also be seen at the 'macule cerulae' site of the bites. The crab louse and their nits may be seen at the root and on the hair shafts, by the naked eye.

Diagnosis

It is ascertained by the recovery of louse and/or nits.

Treatment

Gamma benzene hexachloride (Lorexane) in 0.1 percent concentration is given for the topical application. It is thoroughly rubbed over the affected skin. Usually, one application is sufficient, but it may be repeated on the third day in case of heavy infestation. Secondary infection may be treated accordingly.

MOLLUSCUM CONTAGIOSUM

Molluscum contagiosum is a viral tumor, caused by a DNA-containing poxvirus. Molluscum contagiosum virus (MCV) is a brick-shaped particle, 300 × 200 × 100 mm in size. It replicates in aggregates within the cytoplasm of the infected cells. Basal cell proliferation and epidermal transit time are increased in infected epidermis.

Clinical Features

Molluscum contagiosum is characterized by dome-shaped, waxy pink papules or nodules 2 to 5 mm in size. Central umblication is its hallmark. Some lesions may attain a size up to 1 cm. They are at first firm, solid, and flesh colored. However, as they mature, they tend to become softened and pearly white in color. Some lesions may suppurate. They are distributed over the face, hands, lower abdomen, and genitalia. The mucous membranes of the lip, tongue, and buccal mucosa may also be affected. The lesions are usually a few, at times they may be multiple. They are asymptomatic. Gigantic lesions of size 1 cm or more, may occasionally develop inflammation. Rarely the lesions may become horny (molluscum contagiosum carnuatum).

The disease is contracted by direct contact with infected skin, and by autoinoculation. It may also be transmitted sexually. It affects children, and young adults. Incubation period ranges from 2 to 3 weeks. Immunosuppression secondary to drugs like corticosteroids, methotraxate, and infection with human immunodeficiency virus (HIV) may predispose to widespread and recalcitrant molluscum contagiosum. It usually runs a self-limiting course of 6 to 9 months, but occasionally the lesions may persist for months or years.

Diagnosis

Pearly-white, dome-shaped papule or nodule with central umblication is distinctive. Diagnosis may be confirmed by incising one of the papules, squashing the contents between two glass slides and staining it with Wright's or Giemsa's stain. Examination under a low power of the microscope reveals ovoid, smooth-walled, homogenous cytoplasmic masses consisting of mature, immature, and incomplete virions along with cellular debris. They measure 25 mm in diameter (Fig. 17.4).

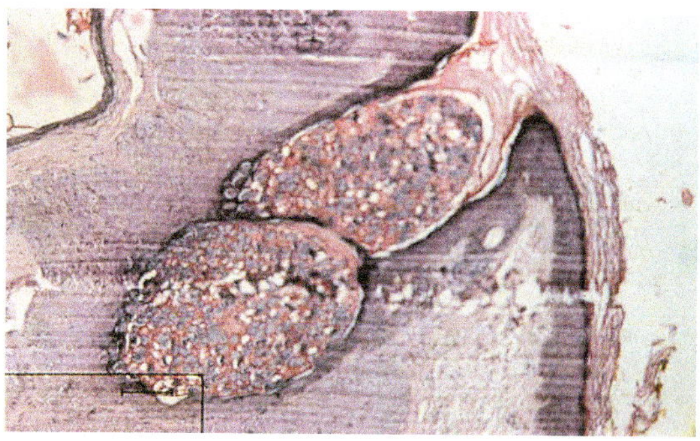

Fig. 17.4: Microscopic examinations

Microscopic examination of hematoxylin eosin-stained section reveals, an acanthoma with downward proliferation of rete ridges, and envelopment by connective tissue to form a deep crater. The cytoplasm of the prickle cell contains numerous small eosinophilic and later basophilic inclusion bodies called molluscum bodies, or Henderson-Patterson bodies. Their bulk compresses the nucleus to the side of the cell. A fully developed lesion depicts a crater near the surface, which extends into the lobules. The crater contains the hyalinized molluscum bodies.

Treatment

The following modalities are useful:

- Removal of the lesion with a sharp curette.
- Cryotherapy with liquid nitrogen or dry ice.
- Electrodesiccation.

FURTHER READING

1. Brown TJ, Yen-Moore A, Tyring SK. An overview of sexually transmitted diseases. Part II. J Am Acad Dermatol 1999; 41: 661-77.
2. Czelusta A, Yen-Moore A, Van der Straten M, Carrasco D, Tyring SK. An overview of sexually transmitted diseases. Part III. Sexually transmitted diseases in HIV-infected patients. J Am Acad Dermatol 2000;43:409-32.
3. Mellanby K. Scabies (2nd ed). Hampton, England: EW classey 1972.
4. Orkin M, Maibach HL, Parish LC et al. Scabies and Pediculosis. Philadelphia: JB Lippincott 1977;1-138.
5. Rosen T, Brown TJ. Cutaneous manifestations of sexually transmitted diseases. Med Clin North Am 1998;82:1081-104.
6. Sehgal VN, Rao TL, Rege VL, Vadiraj SN. Scabies of incidence and treatment method. Int J Dermatol 1972;11:106-11.
7. Sehgal VN, Rege VI, Sehgal N, Kharangate VN, Mascarenhas MF. Epidemiological and clinical pattern of genital lesions. Int J Dermatol 1976; 15: 595-9.
8. Sehgal VN, Gangwani OP. Genital fixed drug eruptions. Genitourin Med 1986; 62:56-8.
9. Sehgal VN, Rege VL, Malik GB. Chronic plasma cell balanitis of zoon. Br J Vener Dis 1973; 49:1986-8.
10. Tariq A, Ross JD. Viral sexually transmitted infections: current management strategies. J Clin Pharm Ther 1999; 24: 409-14.

Chapter 18

Genitoulcerative Diseases

INTRODUCTION

Genitoulcerative diseases (GUD) sores are commonly encountered in practice. Invariably they are of venereal origin, but non-venereal lesions may also occur. The history sexual intercourse is usually positive but in some, misleading history may be contradictory to the clinical picture. By and large and clinical diagnosis of these lesions is easy, but a few may create a diagnostic problem. It is, therefore, relevant to review the salient clinical features and essential office diagnostic procedures of such lesions. Although it may appear a repetition, yet it is vital to make the subject comprehensive. The following conditions form the differential diagnosis of the genital sores (Table 18.1).

CHANCROID

The characteristic lesions are multiple, superficial, painful, dirty, necrotic ulcers. The ulcers are of varying sizes and shapes. The edges of the lesions are undermined, and surrounded by a narrow zone of erythema and edema. The floor is covered by dirty necrotic tissue. They are non-indurated, tender, and bleed on touch. They are usually associated with an unilateral, uniocular and tender swelling. The surface is taut and erythematous in the earlier stages. Later it may show fluctuation. It may burst to form a sinus. The diagnosis is confirmed by the demonstration of *Haemophilus ducreyi* from smears stained with Gram's stain, prepared from a clean ulcer or an aspirate from a bubo.

PRIMARY CHANCRE

A typical ulcer is single, painless, well-defined, clean with raw exuding surface. It is non-tender and markedly indurated, like a button glued to the skin or mucous membrane (see Fig. 8.3). Variations of the classical lesion may be noticed in some patients. Occasionally, ulcers may be multiple with a greyish-white pellicle on the surface. It may become painful due to secondary infection or invasion by *Haemophilus ducreyi*. It is usually accompanied by bilateral inguinal lymphadenopathy. The latter is recognized by their characteristic clinical features. They are multiple, non-tender, discrete, firm and mobile glands. The diagnosis is established by the demonstration of *Treponema pallidum* under the dark-ground microscope by the regular wet preparation or by the direct fluorescent technique. The material for the test is obtained from the ulcer and/or the inguinal glands.

CONDYLOMATA LATA

It is a well-recognized lesion of the secondary stage of syphilis, characterized by broad-based, flat-topped, grayish-white, moist, indurated, fleshy papules. The history of sexual intercourse, a primary

Table 18.1: Differential diagnosis of genital sores

Donovanosis (Granuloma inguinale)	*Lymphogranuloma Venereum (LGV)*	*Chancroid*	*Primary chancre*
1. Causative agent: *Calymmatobacterium granulomatis*	*Chlamydia trachomatis (subtypes L1, L2, L3)*	*Haemophilus ducreyi*	*Treponema pallidum*
2. Incubation period: 3 to 90 days	6 to 42 days	2 to 7 days	9 to 90 days
3. Morphology: Fleshy, exuberant, beefy-red, non-indurated, non-tender, single elevated, granulomatous ulcer, profuse bleeding on touch, recalcitrant without treatment	Transient, herpetiform, spontaneously healing vesicular lesions	Necrotic, small superficial dirty multiple tender, non-indurated ulcers with under-mined edges surrounded by erythematous halo. Dwarf, giant, follicular serpiginous and phagendenic are its variants.	A clean button-like markedly indurated, non-tender, single ulcer which oozes serum. Heals within 4-6 weeks even without treatment
4. Inguinal lymphadenitis: Conspicuously absent.	Inguinal syndrome, with a tendency to suppurate and form multiple fis-tulae in males, is its hall-mark and anorectal ulceration and hyper-plasia in females	Inguinal bubo, if present is unilateral unilocular fluctu-ant and tender, with over lying tout and erythematous skin	Characteristic rubbery disc-rete, mobile, non-tender and bilateral
5. Site of affliction: Moist stratified squa-mous epithelium is the prime target	Lymphatics of the groins, genital and rectum are affected	Undersurface of prepuce its orifice and shaft penis, glans penis, coronal sulcus and frenum less frequently, in female, chiefly the labia majora, fourchette and labia minora	Coronal Sulcus, under sur-face of the prepuce, glans penis and preputial orifice, the labia majora and minora, clitoris fourchettee cervix and the vagina in females. May be extragenital in both.
6. Constitutional symptoms: Absent	Marked, characterised by fever, malaise arthralgia and are present either before or along with its local mani-festations	Absent	Generally absent
7. Elephantiasis: Uncommon, if present, secondary to healing ulcers	Common, ulcer are its secondary feature	Absent	Absent
8. Strictures: Uncommon, if present, are confined to anus	Common and affect the rectum	Absent	Absent
9. Diagnosis: Tissue smears: Donovan bodies in mononuclear cells in Giemsa-stained tissue-	Unhelpful	Scrape smear: Demonstration of gram-negative rods with bipolar condensation of chromatin,	Dark-field examination Demonstration of brilliantly bright spiral, sluggishly motile, Treponema pallidum

Contd

Contd

Donovanosis (Granuloma inguinale)	*Lymphogranuloma Venereum (LGV)*	*Chancroid*	*Primary chancre*
Donovanosis smears and tissue sect-ions is diagnostic	Lymphogranuloma	Chancroid (Granuloma inguinale) arranged in parallel short-chains (school of fish) is diagnostic	Primary chancre Venereum (LGV) from oozing serum, in dark-ground microscopy is confirmatory
10. Blood investigations: Inconclusive	Hyperglobulinemia with reversal of albumin globulin ratio, raised erythrocyte sedimentation rate and leucocytosis are complementary	Inconclusive	
11. Serological test: Unrewarding	The demonstration of four-fold or a greater rise in microimmuno-fluorescent antibody with immunefluorescent type 1, 2, 3 strains of Chlamydia trachomatis confirms the diagnosis		Reagin tests: positive/reactive flocculation VDRL CFT tests Specific tests: TPI, FTA-abs, TPHA and RP-CFT

chancre, the occurrence of syphilids on other parts of the body, and finding of *Treponema pallidum* from the lesions help in the diagnosis. Standard and specific serological tests for syphilis are reactive.

GUMMATOUS ULCER

It has a punched out appearance with clear-cut vertical edges, and a slough-covered base. These lesions have a tendency to central healing and peripheral spread, giving a horse-shoe or a polycyclic appearance. A history of syphilis along with its other evidence may be found. A reactive serology and a favorable response to syphilitic therapy may be contributory.

HERPES PROGENITALIS

These lesions are characterized by the formation of small, vesicles, arranged in groups, over an erythematous background. They may rupture to form multiple, superficial, painful, erosions which may get infected. It is usually preceded by burning sensation. The recurrence of the lesions is the hallmark of the disease. The diagnosis may be supplemented by the demonstration of rounded and ballooned cells in smear containing viral inclusions.

TRAUMATIC ULCERS

It is characterized by a superficial abrasion or a cut which may get secondary infected—form a painful, dirty erosion or an ulcer, resembling chancroid. Granuloma pyogenicum may occur, though rarely. It is a rounded vascular tumor of bright-red color. It is pedunculated and shows blanching on pressure (Fig. 18.1). It may be associated with a unilateral bubo. The history of trauma or abrasion during coitus is usual.

FIXED DRUG ERUPTIONS

The initial eruption may be an erythematous, edematous macule, which may turn into a vesicle or bulla. A superficial erosion or a painful ulcer may be found. The recurrence of the condition on re-exposure to the drug, followed by a remnant hyperpigmented macule at the site (fixed) is the hallmark of the disease.

LYMPHOGRANULOMA VENEREUM

It may resemble herpes progenitalis usually a small, superficial, evanescent herpetiform lesion, which may turn into a nodule or an ulcer. Constitutional symptoms such as fever, malaise or arthralgia may be associated. The diagnosis may be confirmed by hypergammaglobinemia, culture, Frei's test and complement-fixation test, in the later stages of the disease.

GRANULOMA INGUINALE

The early lesion may be a papule, a subcutaneous nodule or an ulcer. The papule is firm and flat-topped, covered by skin or mucous membrane. It may erode to form an ulcer of varying sizes. The ulcer is relatively painless, bright-red in color, soft, velvety with a wavy or serpiginious outline, covered by a film of serosanguinous or a thin translucent parchment-like crust. The ulcers may show variations and may be fleshy, exuberant, hypertrophic, sclerotic or destructive. The diagnosis is confirmed by the recovery of *Donovania granulomatis* (the Donovan body) from the tissue smears.

LICHEN PLANUS

It is recognized by greyish-white dots, streaks or a plaque, which stand prominently over the mucous membrane and/or skin (Fig. 18.2). Vesicles or bullae forming erosions or ulcers may rarely be seen. The diagnosis is usually easy, when the genital lesions are a part accompaniment of lichen planus at other sites. The confirmation of the diagnosis may be possible by histology.

LICHEN NITIDUS

The classic lesions are skin colored, shiny, flat-topped, discrete, multiple papules of pin-head size (Fig. 18.3). The eruptions are asymptomatic. Usually the patient reports for cosmetic reasons. The diagnostic clinch lies in characteristic histopathology.

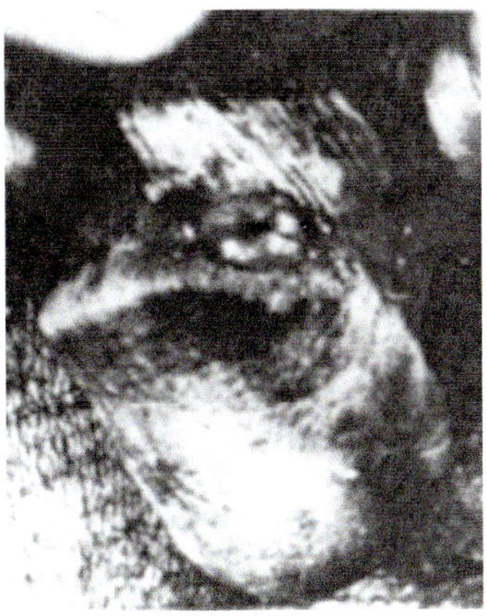

Fig. 18.1: Traumatic ulcer: Granuloma pyogenicum.

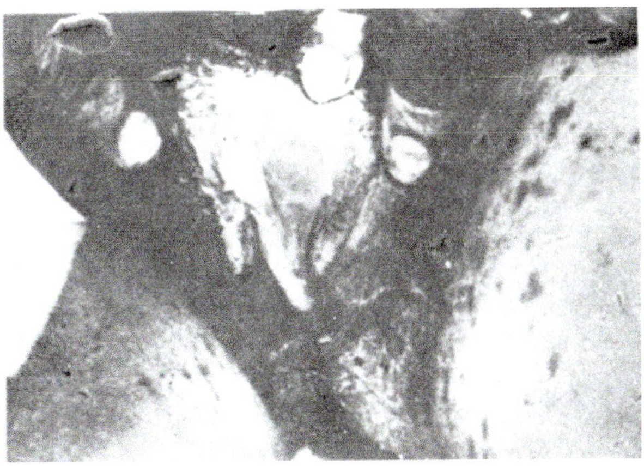

Fig. 18.2: Lichen planus of the vulva

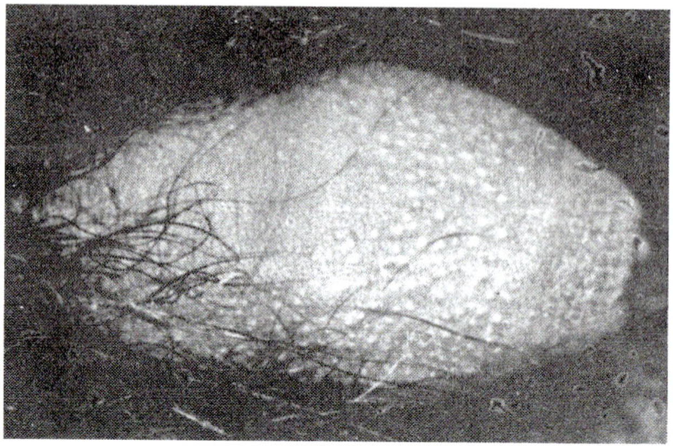

Fig. 18.3: Lichen nitidus, skin colored, shiny flat-topped discrete, multiple, papules on the shaft of the penis

BALANITIS (VULVITIS) CIRCUMSCRIPTA PLASMA CELLULARIS

The lesions in this condition are circumscribed, persistent, moist, soft, granulomatous and velvety. The bright-red color is striking (Figs 18.4A and B). The inguinal lymphadenopathy is conspicuous by its absence. The condition clinically resembles erythroplasia of Queyrat, but the microscopic pathology determines the diagnosis. The dense plasma cells infiltrate in the dermis with conspicuous dilated dermal blood vessels, are the diagnostic features of the disease.

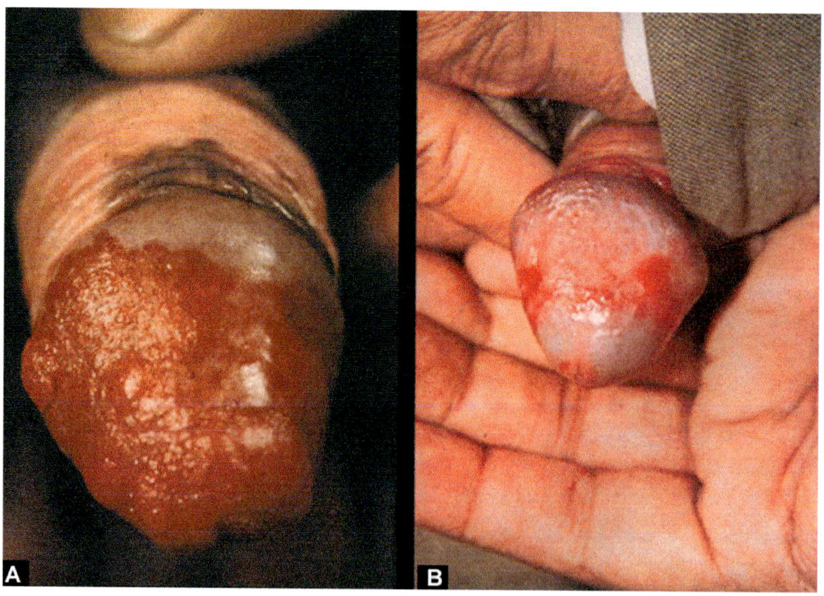

Figs 18.4A and B: Balanitis circumscripta plasma cellularis on the under surface of the prepuce (*Courtesy:* Dr VN Sehgal, et al Birt-J Vener Dis Vener 1974;49: 86).

ERYTHROPLASIA OF QUEYRAT

The clinical features are similar to balanitis (vulvitis) circumscripta plasma cellularis. The histology, however, confirms the diagnosis—it presents as squamous cell carcinoma *in situ*.

EPITHELIOMA

It may present as a papule, nodule, warty or fungating growth. The ulcer, when present, has classical features of malignancy. Initially, it is non-tender, progressive, well-defined, firm with rolled margins, and bleeds easily on touch (Fig. 18.5). The inguinal lymphadenopathy may be a feature in the late stages. Confirmation of the diagnosis is made by finding the features of squamous cell carcinoma histologically.

Other lesions such as tuberculosis, filariasis, cutaneous amebiasis and psoriasis may also be considered, though their occurrence is rare.

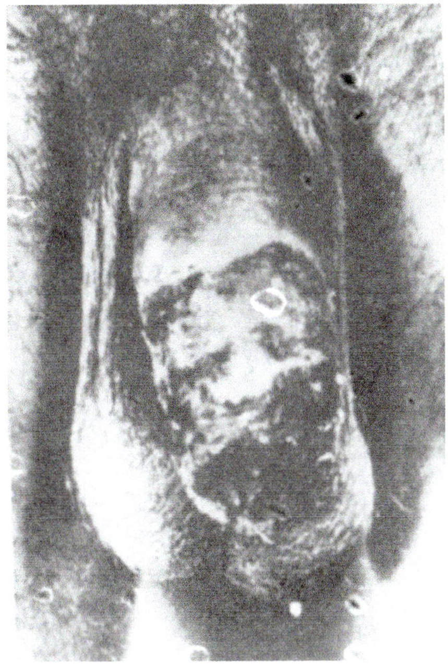

Fig. 18.5: Epithelioma: Malignant ulcer

FURTHER READING

1. Rawlins S. Nonviral sexually transmitted infections. J Obstet Gynecol Neonatal Nurs 2001;30:324-31.

Chapter 19

Nonvenereal Treponematoses

Nonvenereal treponematoses include: yaws, pinta, endemic syphilis, and bejel.

YAWS

Yaws is a nonvenereal chronic contagious disease of tropics and subtropics caused by *Treponema pertenue.*

Epidemiology

It is essentially a disease of children, but may also occur in adults. It occurs in tropics and subtropics. It was endemic in Western Samoa, Haiti, Indonesia, Malaysia, Thailand, Yugoslavia and in some parts of India. It is linked with poor living standard and hygiene-overcrowding, the common use of unclean beds and utensils and lack of soap. Other factors like temperature and altitude, rainfall and humidity may contribute or modify its clinical features. Recent mass treatment campaign, has considerably reduced the prevalence of yaws in the aforesaid endemic areas. It is, however, interesting to find the resurgence of sexually acquired syphilis amongst the younger generation in these countries. It is attributed to considerable decline in immunity against *Treponema pallidum.*

Etiology

It is caused by *Treponema pertenue.* It was discovered by Castellani in 1905. Its morphology is indistinguishable from *Treponema pallidum.*

Pathogenesis

It is transmitted by direct contact with an infected person. The portal of entry is through an apparently healthy skin. It is probable that flies and insects may also transmit the disease. The primary histological changes are in the corium characterized by dense granulomatous infiltrate comprising neutrophils, lymphocytes, histiocytes with predominance of plasma cells. The epidermis shows acanthosis, papillomatosis, edema, microabscesses formation due to migration of neutrophils, in the early stage. The treponemes are demonstrable in the epidermis between the epidermal cells. The secondary lesions are similar to that of primary. The late yaws lesions resemble that of late syphilis with minimal or no change in the blood vessels. The ulcerative lesions of late yaws may additionally have pseudoepitheliomatous hyperplasia and fibrosis of the corium in the healing lesions of the yaws. The changes in the bones are characterized by rerefaction and new bone formation.

Classification

Its clinical course may be divided into an early yaws comprising primary and secondary stages, and late yaws comprising tertiary stage. The early yaws is infective and may last from three to five years. It may be punctuated by latency and relapse. The late yaws is non-infective and may appear three to five years after infection. It is also marked by long periods of latency.

EARLY YAWS

Incubation Period

It is variable. The lesions usually appear after an interval of two to eight weeks.

Clinical Features

Primary Stage

It starts with an erythematous rounded papule, mother yaw at the site of inoculation. It is usually single, but multiple primary lesions may occur. The papule rapidly changes into a nodule and assumes a granulomatous or papillomatous appearance with a diameter of 2-5 cm. The lesions may ulcerate (Figs 19.1 and 19.2) and may become painful due to secondary infection. It may involute by scar formation. It may be accompanied by painless regional lymphadenopathy. The lesicn occurs usually on the exposed parts namely the legs, the feet, the arms and the face. The scalp or the buttocks may also get affected.

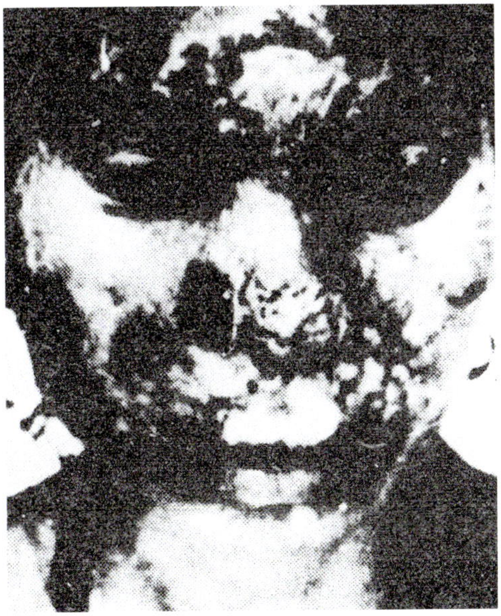

Fig. 19.1: Yaws (*Courtesy:* Dr (Mrs) K Vimlabai)

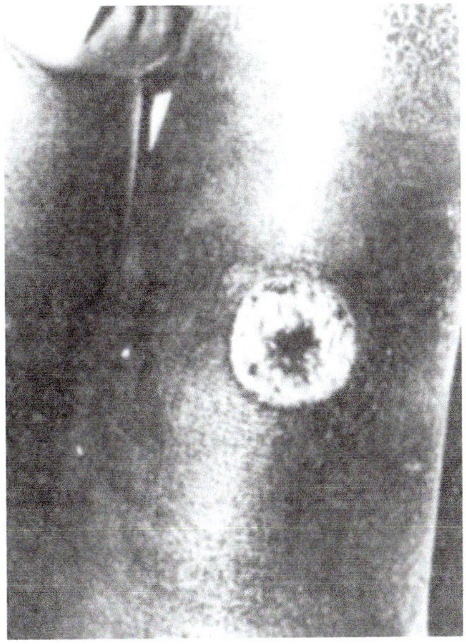

Fig. 19.2: Yaws (*Courtesy:* Dr G Elste Brit J Vener Dis, 1976;52:206)

Secondary Stage

It affects the skin and the bones.

Skin: The morphology of the skin lesions resembles the secondary stage of syphilis. They usually start three to six weeks after the occurrence and/or involution of the mother yaws (Figs 19.3 to 19.5).

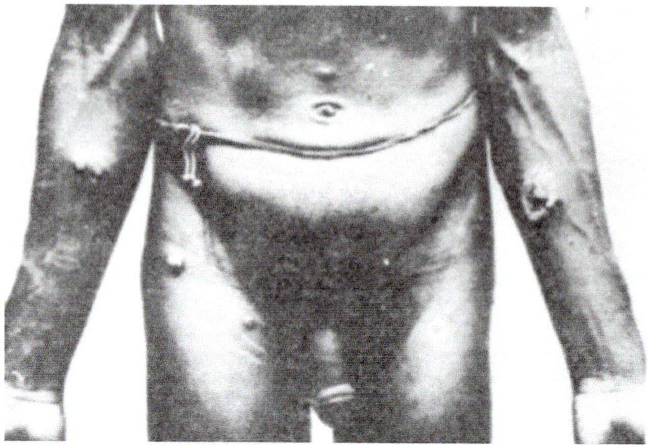

Fig. 19.3

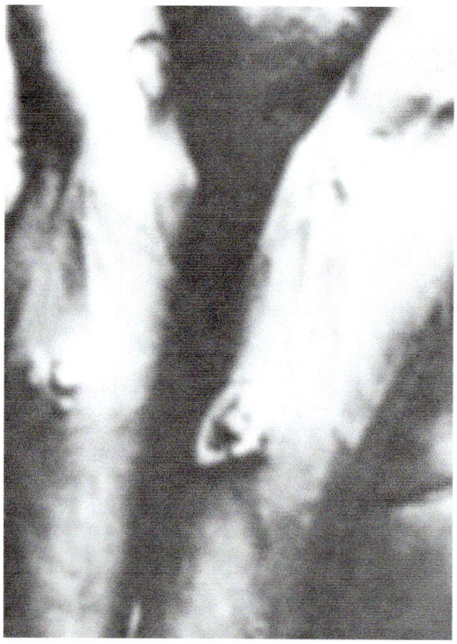

Fig. 19.4

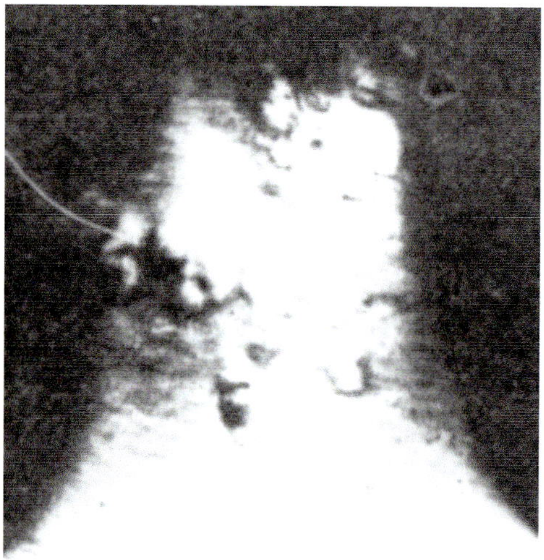

Fig. 19.5

Figs 19.3 to 19.5: Multiple, large hypertrophic erythematous, moist or dry granulomatous papules—*framboesioma* (*Courtesy*: Dr PN Rangiah, Chennai)

The lesions may be of various types such as macules, maculopapules, papules, papulosquamous, micropapules, umbilicated papules, plaques and nodules. The classic lesions of secondary yaws, however, are multiple, large, hypertrophic, erythematous, moist or dry granulomatous papules—*framboesioma*. The lesions usually heal without scarring. They may occur anywhere over the body, but the sites of predilection are moist surfaces such as the groins, the perineal) region, the axillae and around the mucocutaneous junctions. The lesions in the later stages may resemble condylomata lata (Fig. 19.6). The lesions on the palms and soles may present as macules, hyperkeratosis or fissures (Fig. 19.7).

Bones: During this stage long as well as short bones of the extremities may show osteoperiostitis, characterized by pain and tenderness of the bones. These lesions usually resolve without any sequelae.

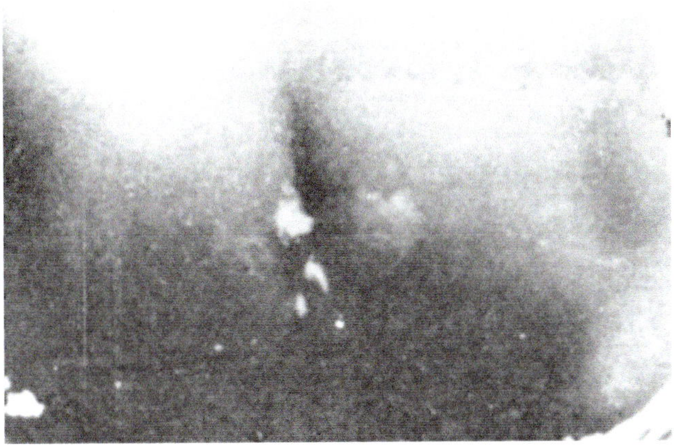

Fig. 19.6: Secondary yaws. Condylomata lata (*Courtesy:* Dr PN Rangiah, Chennai)

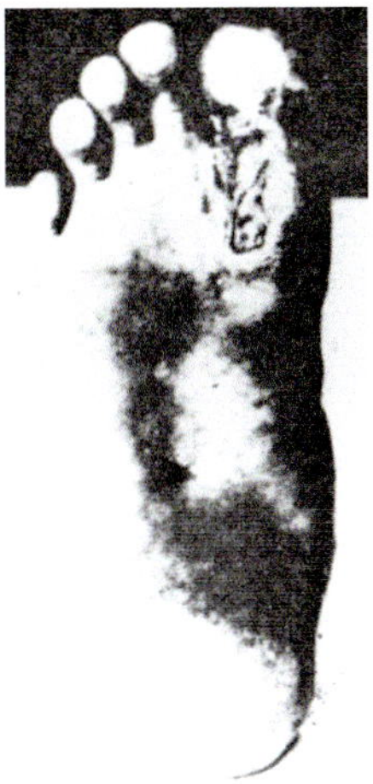

Fig. 19.7: Crab yaws. Modified papillomatous ulcerated plaques on the soles (*Courtesy:* Dr PN Rangiah, Chennai)

Skiagram may reveal areas of rarefaction and new bone formation. In children, occasionally dactylitis may be seen. The upper nasal processes of the maxilla may be hypertrophic due to osteoperiostitis, manifesting as *gondou.*

LATE YAWS

Clinical Features

Late yaws usually occurs from three to five years or more after the infection. The skin, subcutaneous tissue and bones are chiefly affected.

Skin: Skin lesions may be of various types, but they mostly resemble gumma of late syphilis.

Nodular/noduloulcerative lesions They may be intracutaneous or subcutaneous. Their size is variable. They usually start as multiple, indurated, non-tender and mobile nodules. Superficial nodules ulcerate to form clear cut large destructive ulcers with dirty yellow slough. It may involve the bone underneath and form destructive bony lesions, specially involving the bones, and cartilages of the nose presenting as gangosa with through and through perforation of the face. These lesions may heal and leave behind tissue paper—scars or contractures.

Lesions may be seen over the palms and soles, characterized by hyperkeratosis, fissuring and patchy ulceration. These lesions resemble the secondary lesions of yaws and may at times be difficult to differentiate. They may heal leaving behind leukomelanoderma of the palms and soles.

Bones: The long bones, the clavicle and the small bones of the hands and feet may show extensive periosteal reaction along with rarefaction and at times osteomyelitis. The overlying skin and subcutaneous tissue may ulcerate, if bony tissue is close to the lesion. The affected bones are painful and tender as in the secondary stage of yaws. Constitutional symptoms such as low grade pyrexia, malaise and generalized lymphadenopathy may be present. The involvement of the joints may either be due to hydroarthrosis or bursitis. There may be formation of subcutaneous, painless, firm swellings around the joints—*juxta-articular nodes.* Usually the large joints of the extremities are the site of affliction (Table 19.1).

Table: 19.1: Clinical features

		Early yaws		*Late yaws*
		Primary	*Secondary*	*Tertiary*
1.	Incubation period	9 to 90 days	6 to 16 weeks after primary	5 to 15 years, after latency
2.	Cutaneous Lesions	'Mother yaw'	'Daughter yaws'	Gummatous ulcer(s)
	Character	Typical framboesioma A reddish, non-tender papulonodule, progresses to crusted erosion, with papillomatous proliferations on granulomatous base satellite lesions may coalesce treponemes abundant.	Disseminated crustopapillomatous eruptions 'Pickled cauliflower' appearance cardinal Circinate lesions with central healing and peripheral expansion and macular, maculosquamous, maculopapular, papular, papulonodular eruptions simulating syphilids Serous discharge rich in treponemes Occasionally only 'Id' eruption 'Crab yaws', modified, tender, papillomatous ulcerated plaque on the sole	Progressively enlarging, painless nodule, that undergoes necrosis and ulceration Well-defined edges, indurated base and floor covered with granulation and yellowish slough Spontaneous healing with keloid formation Palmoplantar hyperkeratosis may accompany
	Symptoms	Pruritic/Asymptomatic	Pruritic	Asymptomatic
3.	Site	Exposed areas, especially lower legs	Disseminated	Extremities, usually legs
4.	Other systems	Associated lymphadenopathy	Constitutional symptoms Lymphadenopathy Skeletal involvement 1. Periostitis and osteitis 2. Bursitis 3. 'Gondou', exostoses of nasal and maxillary bones.	Skeletal involvement, gummatous/non-gummaotus The former is firm fibrous, juxta-articular nodule, that ulcerates to form gummatous ulcer, while latter shows periostitis, with cortical thickening; Sabre tibia, boomerang legs and gangosa (destructive ulcerative rhinopharyngitis)
5.	Course	Spontaneous resolution (2 to 9 months)	Spontaneous resolution, with residual pigmentation	Heals with scarring, may form keloids

'Attenuated', modified, less florid yaws in areas under mass treatment campaigns

Diagnosis

It is made by the history of residence in an endemic areas, contact with an infective case, the characteristic clinical manifestations of the disease and the demonstration of *T. pertenue* under the dark-ground microscope by the regular wet preparations or by the direct fluorescent technique. The material for the test is obtained from primary or secondary lesions or from the enlarged lymph glands. The organisms are recognized by its morphology, motility or fluorescence. Reactive standard as well as specific serological tests for syphilis are diagnostic. These tests usually take about six weeks to become reactive after the appearance of the primary lesions of yaws. They may remain reactive throughout the course of the disease though quantitatively the titers may show a decline in late or burnt out cases. Radiological examination of bones usually shows periosteal reaction with rarefaction and necrosis specially in late cases (Table 19.2).

Table 19.2: Laboratory diagnosis of yaws

	Early yaws		*Late yaws*
	Primary	*Secondary*	*Tertiary*
1. Dark-ground for *T. pallidum* subspecies *pertenue*	Positive	Positive	Negative
2. Fluorescent microscopy (Fluorescein conjugated anti-*T. pallidum* subspecies *pertenue* monoclonals)	Positive	Positive	Negative
3. Serological tests (specific and non-specific)	Reactive	Reactive	Reactive
4. Histopathology	1. Dense dermal granulomatous infiltrate comprising plasma cells and lymphocytes. A few neutrophils and histiocytes. 2. Vascular alteration minimal 3. Treponemes on silver impregnation	1. Dense dermal granulomatous infiltrate comprising plasma cells and lymphocytes. Few neutrophils and histiocytes. 2. Vascular alteration minimal 3. Treponemes on silver impregnation	1. Intense dermal infiltrate comprising epithelioid cells, giant cells, lymphocytes and fibroblasts. Few plasma cells and histiocytes 2. Caseation necrosis at the center 3. Treponemes, only occasional

Treatment

Penicillin is the antibiotic of choice. Long-acting repository penicillin administered in adequate doses are sufficient to control the disease. Benzathine penicillin (Penidure LA 24) in the dosage of 1.2 mega units is adequate for the treatment of yaws (Table 19.3). The same dosage are used in treatment of contact. Several other alternative antibiotics are now available for its treatment in penicillin-sensitive patients. Erythromycin and tetracycline may be used in the same dosage as for syphilis.

PINTA

Pinta is a nonvenereal treponemal disease, characterized by erythematous, pigmented and depigmented eruptions over the exposed parts of the body.

Table 19.3: Evolution of treatment

		1952	*1955*	*1960*	*1982*
1.	Drug	PAM*	PAM*	PAM*	Benzathine penicillin
2.	Treatment Active cases				
	Adults	1.2 million units, single dose	1.2 million units, single dose	1.2 million units, single dose	1.2 million units single dose
	Children	Appropriate lower dosage	0.6 million units (< 15 yr)	0.6 million units (< 15 yr)	0.6 million units (< 10 yr)
3.	Contacts	Half the (dose adminis-tered to active cases	Half the dose	vHalf the dose	Same as for active disease
4.	Control policy	Nil	TMT** (prevalence > 10%) JMT*** (prevalence 5-10%) SMT**** (prevalence < 5%)	TMT** (prevalence > 10%) JMT*** (prevalence 5-10%) SMT**** (prevalence < 5%)	TMT** (prevalence > 10%) JMT*** (prevalence 5-10%) SMT**** (prevalence < 5%)

PAM* : Procaine penicillin in 2% aluminium monostearate
TMT** : Total mass treatment : Entire population
JMT*** : Juvenile mass treatment : All contacts and prepubertal children
SMT**** : Selective mass treatment : Only household and obvious contacts

Epidemiology

The disease is of rare occurrence. It is endemic in central and northern parts of America and some parts of Africa. Only stray cases of the disease have been reported from India. It affects both males and females. It is mainly a disease of children. The disease occurs amongst under-privileged, unhygienic and poor sections of the society.

Etiology

The disease is caused by *Treponema carateum*, which is indistinguishable morphologically from *T. pallidum.*

Pathogenesis

The reservoir of infection is an infected person. The disease is transmitted from an infected individual to a healthy one either by direct skin-to-skin contact or through flies. The organisms mainly involve the skin and subcutaneous tissue. The histopathological changes are similar to that of acquired syphilis.

Incubation Period

It may last for several months.

Clinical Features

They are characterized by the appearance of desquamating erythematous patch, *pintids,* on the exposed parts of the body such as the legs, the arms and the face. Three to five months later multiple, erythematous, scaly lesions appear around the earlier lesions. They may later become coppery-red or brown in color leaving behind greyish or black-colored patches. It is followed by the appearance of depigmented or ivory-white lesions. Some of the lesions may stop short of depigmentation to form hypochromia or dyschromia of the lesions. These changes may take several years to appear from its inception. Hyperkeratosis of the palms and soles along with the juxta-articular nodes may be seen. Aortitis and aneurysm of the ascending aorta may also occur. In some cases the bones may be involved.

Diagnosis

It is made by the clinical features and confirmed by the demonstration of *Treponema carateum* from the early lesions. It is complemented by the reactive standard as well as specific serological tests for syphilis.

Treatment

Penicillin is the drug of choice. The long-acting repository penicillins such as PAM and benzathine penicillin (Penidure LA 12) in recommended dosage of 1.2 mega units are adequate for its treatment. The same dose may, however, be useful for its mass eradication campaign.

ENDEMIC SYPHILIS

Endemic syphilis is a nonvenereal treponematosis, occurring in primitive communities, caused by an organism which is morphologically indistinguishable from *Treponema pallidum.*

Epidemiology

It is endemic in some parts of Africa. It was present in Europe, Yugoslavia, Palestine, Balkans and USSR, but it has now been eradicated in these countries by mass eradication campaigns. Gradually venereal syphilis is replacing endemic syphilis in these areas.

Clinical features and treatment are similar to Bejel (*vide infra*).

BEJEL

Bejel, like endemic syphilis is also a nonvenereal treponematosis.

Epidemiology

The disease is prevalent in the Middle East, Gulf and African countries. It is the disease of poor, underpriviledged and unhygienic individuals. Overcrowding contributes to its propagation. It is a disease of children and affects both males and females.

Etiology

The disease is caused by *Treponema pallidum.*

Pathogenesis

The infection is transmitted from the infected individual to a healthy one by skin-to-skin contact. It may also occur through drinking in common utensils or by fomites. It affects the skin, mucous membranes and the bones, but its transplacental transmission is unknown. Its pathology is similar to that of acquired syphilis.

Incubation Period

It varies from a few months to years.

Clinical Features

The disease is usually devoid of primary stage while the lesions of secondary stage resemble that of acquired syphilis. The characteristic lesions, however, are generalized papules, annular and papulosquamous eruptions. The papules at the moist areas may get hypertrophied to form lesions similar to *condylomata lata* at the genitals and perianal regions. The mucous membrane may get involved to form grayish-white mucous patches similar to that seen in the secondary stage of acquired syphilis. The involvement of larynx and pharynx may give rise to sore throat and hoarseness of voice. The involvement of the bones may cause severe nocturnal pains due to periostitis. The disease may pass on to the tertiary stage after a variable latent period. Gummatous lesions involving the skin, the subcutaneous tissue and the bones characterize the tertiary stage similar to late acquired syphilis. But unlike the latter the involvement of viscera, cardiovascular and nervous system is not known.

Diagnosis

The disease is identified by clinical features. It is, however, confirmed by demonstrating *T. pallidum* by the dark ground examination. Standard and specific serological tests for syphilis are reactive as in syphilis.

Treatment

Penicillin is the treatment of choice. Its dosage depends upon the age of the patient. In infants and children the dosage is 0.3 to 0.6 mega units, while in adults it is 1.2 mega units of long-acting repository penicillin like PAM and benzathine (Penidure LA 12) given in a single dose. The same dose may be useful for its mass eradication.

FURTHER READING

1. Anonymous. Expert committee on venereal infections and treponematoses. Fifth report, World Health Organization Technical Report Series No 190, Geneva; World Health Organization 1960.
2. Anonymous. Endemic treponematoses in the 1980's (editorial). Lancet 1983;2:551-2.
3. Brown ST. Therapy for non-venereal treponematoses: review of the efficacy of penicillin and consideration of alternatives. Rev Infect Dis 1985;7: 318-26.
4. Engelkens HJ, Vuzevski VD, Stolz E. Nonvenereal treponematoses in tropical countries. Clin Dermatol 1999; 17:143-52.
5. Engelkens HJH, Judanarso JJ, Oranja AP, Vuzevski VD, Niemel PL, van der Sluis JJ et al. Endemic treponematoses Part I. Yaws. Int J Dermatol 1991;30:77-83.
6. Fludson FH. Non-venereal Syphilis. Livingston 1958.
7. Hudson FH, Christian HA. Treponematoses. New York: Oxford University Press 1946.
8. Maier H, Cesaire R, Bera O, Kerob-Bauchet B, Ould Amar AK, Desbois N, et al. The role of yaws in the serologic screening of treponematoses in blood donors in Martinique. Transfus Clin Biol 2001;8:403-9.
9. Meheus A. Integration of yaws control and primary health care. Rev Infect Dis 1985;7:284-8.
10. Perine PL, Nelson JW, Lewis JO, Liska S, Hunter EF, Larsen SA, et al. New technologies for use in the surveillance and control of yaws. Rev Infect Dis 1985;7:295-9.
11. Sehgal VN, Jain S, Bhattacharya SN, Thappa DM. Yaws control/eradication. Int J Dermatol 1994;33:16-20.
12. Sehgal VN. Leg ulcers caused by yaws and endemic syphilis. Clin Dermatol 1990;8:166-74.
13. Zahara A. Yaws in south East Asia: an overview. Rev Infect Dis 1985;7:245-50.

Chapter 20

Genital Warts

INTRODUCTION

Warts are benign epidermal proliferations, caused by infection with human papilloma virus (HPV). Its association with various carcinomas has been recently recognized.

The papilloma viruses are members of the family Papovaviridae. It contains double-stranded, circular, supercoiled DNA enclosed in an icosahedral capsid made up of 72 capsomers. The virion has a molecular weight of 5 × 106 daltons. The virus has no envelop, and is resistant to freezing, and dessication. The DNA genome of papilloma virus has 8000 base pairs and the capsid diameter is 55 nm. Serologic typing, as applied to some other viruses, is not useful for HPV. Therefore, DNA hybridization has been used as a means of separating different HPVs. Viruses that hybridize by less than 50 percent with other known types are classified as a new type. To date 55 HPV types have been identified. Many of these types have significant clinicopathologic correlation with genital wart (Table 20.1).

Table 20.1: Clinicopathologic correlation

Clinical types of wart		*Types of HPV*
Genital warts	:	6, 11, 16, 18, 30, 31, 32, 42, 43, 51 to 55
Cervical carcinoma	:	16, 18, 31, 32, 34, 39, 42, 48, 51 to 54

The transmission of HPV occurs by close contact with an infected person. Small breaks in the skin are necessary to inoculate HPV. Autoinoculation is responsible for the local spread of the warts. Many factors are responsible in the infectivity of HPV, including the number of viral particles, the degree and duration of the exposure and the host's defence against HPV infection. Cell-mediated immunity is important in the host defence against HPV.

Genital warts They may be either hyperplastic, sessile (papular); verruca vulgaris like or flat warts.

- *Hyperplastic* They express as single or multiple vegetative lesions. The latter are formed by multiple confluent soft pinkish or grayish white papillomatous projections. They may occasionally proliferate to form a cauliflower mass. The lesions are usually seen in warm and moist areas and are usually localised to the inner surface of the prepuce, frenulum, coronal sulcus, (Figs 20.1A and B) glans penis or external urinary meatus, perianal region (Fig. 20.2). In females, it occupies vaginal introitus (Figs 20.3 and 20.4) inner aspect of vulva, vestibule, and vagina.

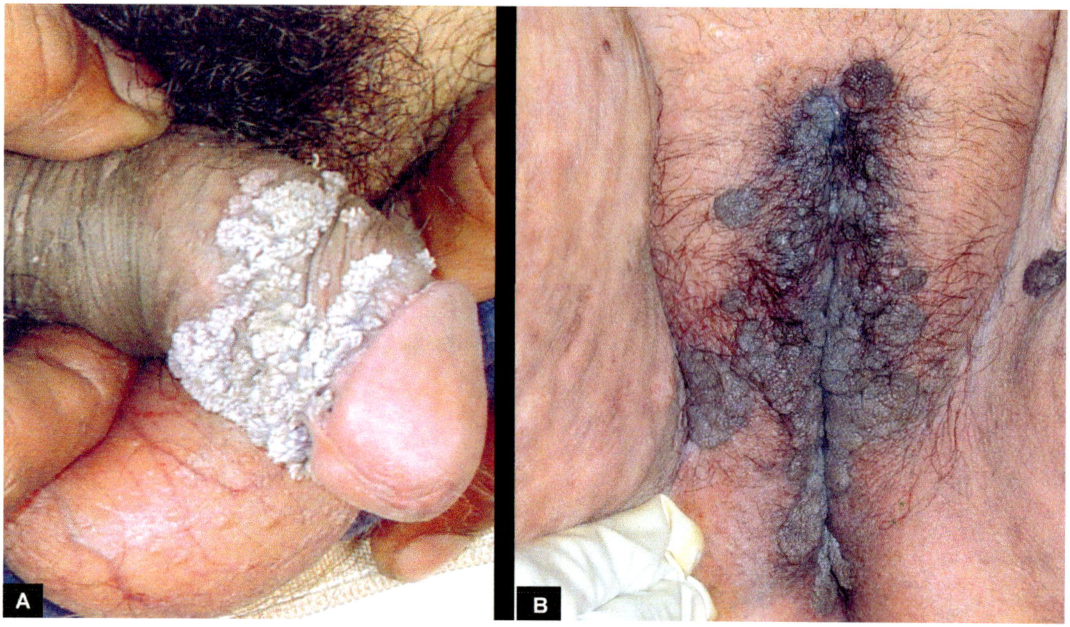

Figs 20.1A and B: Condylomata acuminata—cauliflower like growth

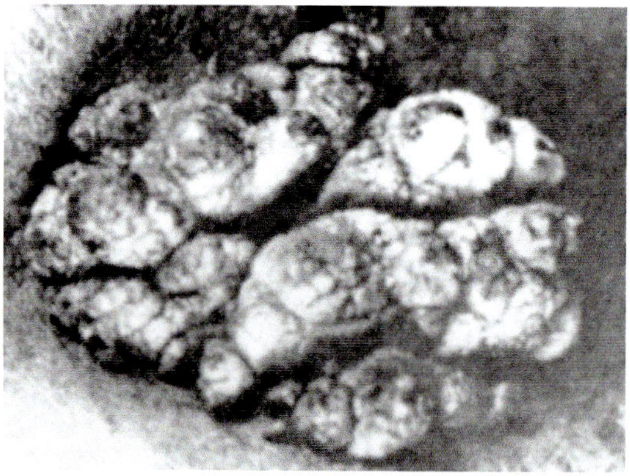

Fig. 20.2: Hyperplastic—cauliflower mass at the anal cleft

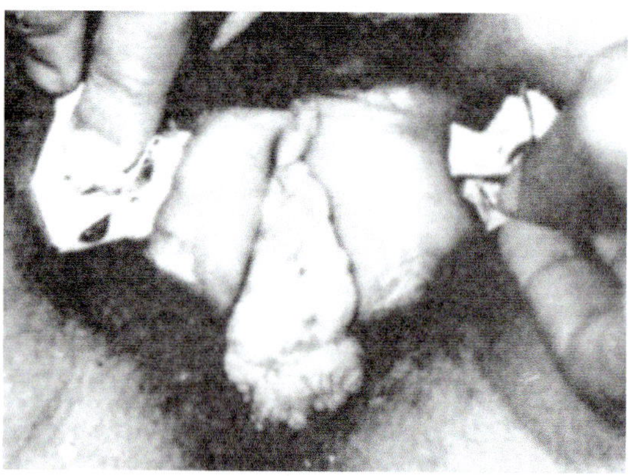

Fig. 20.3: Hyperplastic—cauliflower mass at vaginal introitus

- *Sessile (papular)* They are usually seen as multiple, small discrete and smooth papules. Shaft of the penis in males and the vulva and/or perianal region in females are its common location (Fig. 20.5).
- *Flat warts* They are seen as white spots with punctation over uterine cervix and are identified on colposcopy. Pap smears may be performed to demonstrate koilocyte.
- *Verruca vulgaris type warts* They are recognized as single or multiple with rough irregular surface, simulating common warts. They affect the shaft of the penis, outer aspect of labia, perineum, pubis, and groin.

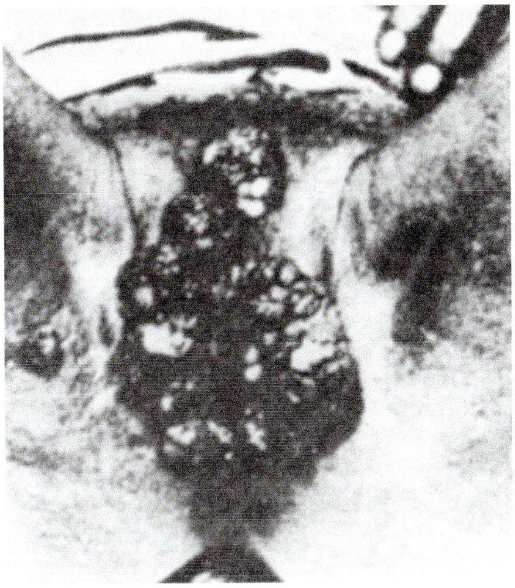

Fig. 20.4: Condylomata acuminata of vulva

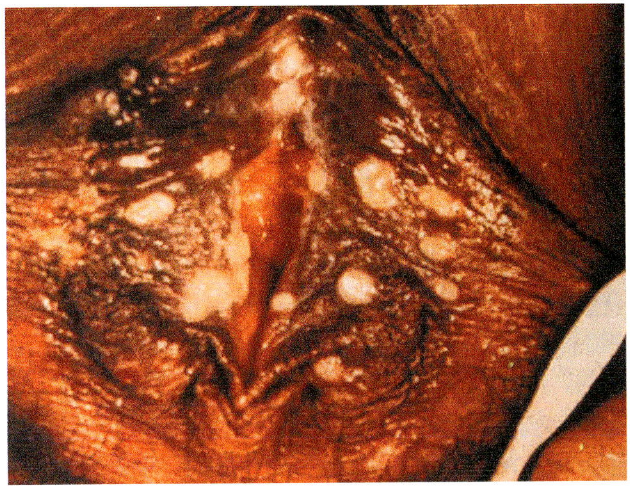

Fig. 20.5: Sessile—multiple, small, discrete smooth surfaced papules

HPV infection and carcinoma The relationship between HPV and human carcinoma has focused mainly on carcinoma of the cervix. Others are the actinically induced squamous cell carcinoma in EBV patient, laryngeal and bronchial carcinoma.

DIAGNOSIS

It is clinical. It may be supplemented by histopathology and detection of HPV.

Microscopic examination of hematoxylin-eosin stained section of common warts reveals: (1) Parakeratosis, (2) Hyperkeratosis, (3) Papillomatosis, (4) Acanthosis. The acanthotic rete ridges tend to point radially towards the center of the lesion, (5) Vacuolated cells, with small basophilic nuclei surrounded by a clear halo and pale cytoplasm (koilocytes) (Fig. 20.6) are found in the upper stratum granulosum. These cells lack keratohyaline granules. The flat warts lack the papillomatosis and parakeratosis seen in common warts. Anogenital warts have marked acanthosis and rete ridges display pseudoepitheliomatous hyperplasia.

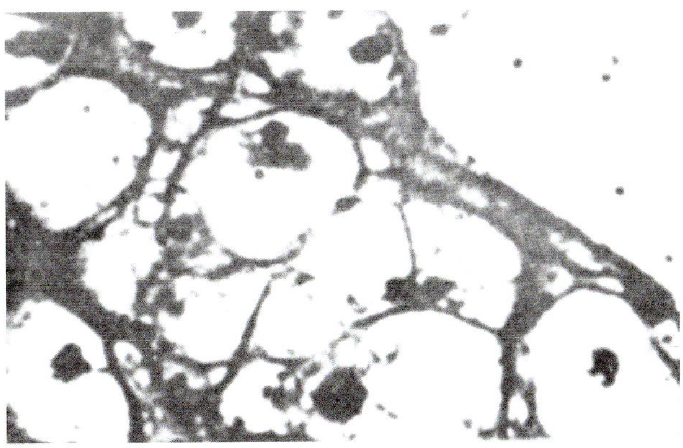

Fig. 20.6: Koilocyte—vacuolated cells, small basophilic nuclei surrounded by a clear halo and pale cytoplasm

Detection of HPV Recent advances in molecular biology have facilitated the detection of HPV DNA within the tissue. The techniques used are:

- Nucleic acid hybridization, which allows identification of specific DNA or RNA sequences.
- Cleavage of DNA by restriction endonucleases.

- DNA cloning by the use of recombinant molecules. Southern blotting is the technique used to identify HPV DNA
- Polymerase chain reaction, which allows the targeted DNA sequence to be enzymatically amplified before southern blotting. It improves the sensitivity of the test. A single molecule of HPV DNA may be detected in 10^5 cells by this techniques.

Table 20.2: Treatment of warts

Types	*Modalities of treatment*	*Newer therapy*
Condylomata acuminata	25 percent podophyllin in compound tincture of benzoin applied every 3rd or 4th day. The surrounding area should be protected by application of vaseline. After the resin has dried, the wart is sprinkled with powder to prevent transfer of podophyllin to apposing skin. Area is washed with water after 3 to 4 hours.	a. Podophyllotoxin 0.5 percent in ethanol applied twice daily for 3 days, every week. b. Intralesional injection of interferon alfa 2β in doses of 1×10^6 IU thrice a week, for 3 weeks. c. 1×10^6 IU/m^2 of interferon alfa 2β, intramuscular or subcutaneous.

TREATMENT

Treatment is outlined in Table 20.2.

FURTHER READING

1. Bentner KR. Human papilloma virus infection. J Am Acad Dermatol 1989; 20:114-23.
2. Bentner KR, Reitano MV, Richwald GA, Wiley DJ. External genital warts report of the American Medical Association Consensus Conference. AMA Expert Panel on External Genital Warts. Clin Infect Dis 1998;27:796-806.
3. Beutner KR, Wiley DJ, Douglas JM, Tyring SK, Fife K, Trofatter K, et al. Genital warts and their treatment. Clin Infect Dis 1999;28:S37-S56.
4. Cobb MW. Human Papilloma virus infection. J Am Acad Dermatol 1990;22:547-66.
5. Maw RD. Treatment of anogenital warts. Dermatol Clin 1998;16:829-34.
6. McMillan A. The management of difficult anogenital warts. Sex Transm Infect 1999;75:192-4.
7. Oriel JD. Natural history of genital warts. Br J Vener Dis 1971;47:1-13.
8. Samarakoon S. Genital warts. Ceylon Med J 1999;44:159-61.
9. Sehgal VN, Koranne RV, Srivastava SB, Gupta MM, Luthra UK. Clinicopathology and immunohistochemistry of genital warts. Int J Dermatol 1988;27:690-4.
10. Sehgal VN, Koranne RV, Srivastava SB. Genital warts: current status. Int J Dermatol 1989;28:75-85.
11. Tariq A, Ross JD. Viral sexually transmitted infections. current management strategies. J Clin Pharm Ther 1999; 24:409-14.
12. Wright T. Genital warts: their etiology and treatment. Nurs Time 1998;94:52-4.

Chapter 21

Behçet's Disease

INTRODUCTION

Behçet's disease (BD) is a multisystem vasculitis that was originally described as comprising recurrent orogenital ulceration and iritis. Since then, the symptom complex has widened and includes arthritis, cutaneous vasculitis and meningoencephalitis. The peak age of onset is in the third decade and both men and women may be affected. The diagnostic criteria, and laboratory markers for BD are not well-established. The disease tends to run a chronic course with interspersed remissions and exacerbations. At times blindness, pulmonary vasculitis, arterial occlusion and ruptured aneurysms may complicate.

CLINICAL FEATURES

1. Recurrent, painful, aphthous ulceration of the oral cavity is cardinal.
2. Genital ulcers resembling those in the mouth; May heal with scarring.
3. Ocular affliction, accompanying or following orogenital ulceration; Conjunctivitis may be an initial feature, however, anterior uveitis with hypopyon is cardinal; Posterior uveitis with vitreous hemorrhage and retinal detachment may complicate, resulting in blindness.
4. Polyarthritis, affecting knees, ankles, wrists, elbows in fifty percent of patients.
5. Erythema nodosum is characteristic; At times acneiform papulonodules and pustules may accompany; Cutaneous hyperirritability (pathergy) is cardinal.
6. Meningoencephalitis, superficial and deep thrombophlebitis psychogenic symptoms, and colonic ulceration may be additional features.

DIAGNOSIS

It is clinical. The International Diagnostic Criteria laid down for the purpose are helpful (Table 21.1).

Table 21.1: Diagnostic criteria for Behçet's disease

Recurrent oral ulceration	:	Minor or major aphthous or herpetiform ulcers observed by physician or reliably reported by patient, recurring at least 3 times in one 12 months period.
Plus 2 of recurrent genital ulceration	:	Aphthous ulceration or scarring observed by physician or reliably reported by patient.
Eye lesion	:	Anterior or posterior uveitis or cells in vitreous, or retinal vasculitis observed by ophthalmologist.
Skin	:	Erythema nodosum observed by physician or reliably reported by patient or acneiform nodules observed by physician in post-adolescent patients not receiving corticosteroid.
Positive pathergy test	:	Read at 48 hours

Table 21.2: Treatment of Behçet's disease

Affliction	*Treatment of choice*	*Alternatives*
1. Oral ulceration	Topical corticosteroids in orabase	Systemic steroids in severe, deep painful ulceration
2. Genital ulceration	Topical corticosteroid	— do —
3. Eye uveitis	Quiescent/healed eye 2 years duration requires no treatment. For active uveitis 1. Topical steroids and mydriatics 2. Systemic steroids, in adequate doses if the disease is severe	Immunomodulators such as azathioprine and cyclosporine
4. Arthritis	Non-steroidal anti-inflammatory drugs	Colchicine, systemic corticosteroid
5. Cutaneous erythema nodosum	a. Non-steroidal anti-inflammatory drugs b. Systemic steroids	Colchicine

TREATMENT

The details are provided in the Table 21.2.

FURTHER READING

1. Anonymous Behcet's disease. Lancet 1989;2:761-2.
2. Anonymous. Criteria for diagnosis of Behcet's disease. International Study Group for Behcet's Disease. Lancet 1990;335:1078-80.
3. Bang D. Clinical spectrum of Behcet's disease. J Dermatol 2001;28:610-3.
4. Barnes CG. Behcet's syndrome-classification criteria. Ann Med Interne (Paris) 1999;150:477-82.
5. Ehrlich GE. Behcet's disease: an update. Compr Ther 1999;25:216-20.
6. Kontogiannis V, Powell RJ. Behcet's disease. Postgrad Med J 2000;76:629-37.
7. Lee LA. Behcet's disease. Semin Cutan Med Surg 2001;20:53-7.
8. Onder M, Gurer MA. The multiple faces of Behcet's disease and its aetiological factors. J Eur Acad Dermatol Venereal 2001;15:126-36.
9. Serdaroglu P. Behcet's disease and the nervous system. J Neurol 1998;245:197-205.
10. Sakane T, Takeno M. Current therapy in Behcet's disease. Skin Therapy Lett 2000;5:3-5.
11. Yaziei H, Yurdakul S, Hamuryndan V. Behcet's disease. Curr Opin Rheumatol 2001;13:18-22.

Chapter 22

HIV/Acquired Immunodeficiency Syndrome (AIDS)

DEFINITIONS

The term acquired immunodeficiency syndrome (AIDS) refers to the most severe clinical manifestations of infection with the human immunodeficiency virus (HIV). The infection persists for life and an individual may develop clinical manifestation defining AIDS after a varying interval of time. This progression to AIDS reflects the gradual deterioration of the host's immune system characterized by the depletion of the CD4 helper/inducer lymphocytes. Soon after the person becomes infected, the number of CD4 lymphocytes begin to drop from its normal value of about 1000 cells per mm^3, at a variable rate of approximately 40 to 80 cells per mm^3, per year. This progressive deterioration of the immune system is initially manifested as generalized lymphadenopathy, diarrhea, and weight loss. The AIDS defining conditions develop when the counts of CD4 lymphocytes fall below 200 per mm^3.

Centre for disease control (CDC) had defined AIDS as a disease indicative of a defect in cell-mediated immunity occurring in a person with no cause for immunodeficiency other than HIV. Now it has incorporated the CD4 lymphocytes counts below 200 per mm^3, in its revised definition. The major diseases that are considered to indicate a defect in cell-mediated immunity and thus define a person as having AIDS are listed in Table 22.1.

However, extensive investigations of infections and immunity may not be possible in developing countries. To overcome these difficulties, World Health Organization (WHO) has suggested a case-

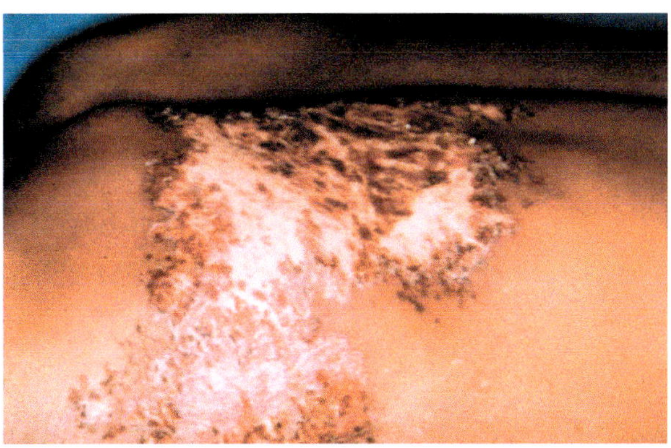

Fig. 22.1: E_1 Herpes-hzoster (HIV) scarring

Table 22.1: AIDS: CDC case definition

Protozoal
Pneumocystis carinii pneumonia (PCP)
Toxoplasmosis of the brain
Cryptosporidiosis with diarrhea > 1 month
Fungal
Candidiasis—esophageal, tracheal, bronchial or pulmonary (oral thrush alone is insufficient for diagnosis of AIDS)
Cryptococcus—meningitis (or other extrapulmonary site)
Viral
Cytomegalovirus (CMV)—retinitis, pneumonitis, colitis, or encephalitis.
Herpes simplex-mucocutaneous disease > 1 month
Progressive multifocal leukoencephalopathy (PML)
Bacterial
Mycobacterium avium intercellular (MAI) or *M. kansasii*-disseminated
Mycobacterium tuberculosis (if extrapulmonary and not confined only to lymph glands in a patient who is HIV antibody positive)
Recurrent non-typhoid Salmonella septicemia (if patient HIV antibody positive)
Tumors
Kaposi's sarcoma : any age if HIV antibody positive : (< 60 if HIV status unknown)
Primary CNS lymphoma
Non-Hodgkin's lymphoma of B cell type (only if patient HIV anti-body positive)
Others
HIV encephalopathy (HIV brain and spinal cord disease/AIDS dementia complex-if patient HIV antibody positive)
HIV wasting syndrome ("slim disease")—if patient HIV antibody positive Lymphoid interstitial pneumonia (LIP) in a child < 13 years

Table 22.2: AIDS: WHO case definition

Major signs

1. Weight loss > 10% of body weight
2. Chronic diarrhea > 1 month
3. Fever > 1 month (intermittent or constant)

Minor signs

1. Persistent cough > 1 month
2. General pruritic dermatitis
3. Recurrent herpes zoster
4. Oropharyngeal candidiasis
5. Chronic progressive and disseminated herpes simplex infection (Fig. 22.1)
6. Generalized lymphadenopathy

definition for use in these developing countries (Table 22.2).

AIDS in an adult is diagnosed if atleast 2 major and 1 minor sign are present in the absence of known cause of immunosuppression.

The etiologic or causative agent of acquired immunodeficiency virus is retrovirus, the human immunodeficiency virus (HIV). It was first isolated in 1983 by Luc Montagnies and his colleagues Francois Barre-Sinoussi and Jean-Claude Chermann from an enlarged lymph node. It was termed lymphadenopathy associated virus. Since then the nomenclature of the virus has been repeatedly changed (Table 22.3).

In 1987, a new retrovirus was identified, it was termed HIV-2 and the original HIV was redesignated HIV-1. The HIV-2 is related to HIV-1 in overall structure and both cause AIDS. However, the pathogenic potential of HIV-2 is not well-established. Furthermore, HIV-2 grows readily in man, monkey, and apes whereas HIV-2 infection occurs predominantly in West Africa whereas HIV-1 infection predominates in east, central, and southern Africa. The salient features of HIV are summarized in Table 22.4.

Table 22.3: Nomenclature of AIDS virus

1983	:	Lymphadenopathy associated virus (LAV)
1984	:	Human T-lymphotropic virus type 3 (HTLV-3)
	:	AIDS related virus (ARV)
1986	:	Human immunodeficiency virus (HIV)
1987	:	HIV-1 and HIV-2

Table 22.4: Salient features of HIV

1. It belongs to the *lentivirus* subfamily of retroviruses.
2. The genetic information is encoded in 2 strands of RNA.
3. The RNA is surrounded by 2 protein coats, namely p 18 and p 24.
4. It possesses a spiked envelope. The outer portion of the spike is called gp 120. The stalk that peneterates the envelope is called gp 41.
5. The 3 genes common to all retroviruses are *gag, pol* and *env.*
   Gag codes for p 24 and p 18.
   Pol codes for the enzyme reverse transcriptase
   Env codes for the synthesis of gp 120 and gp 41.
6. It also contains nonstructural genes *tat, art, 3'orf. Tat* is essential for viral replication and acts as a transactivating factor, acting both on transcription and post-transcriptional modification of all viral proteins.
   Art acts to enhance the synthesis of viral structural proteins by promoting active translation of viral mRNA.
7. HIV infects cells bearing CD4 receptors. gp 120 virus projection bind to CD4 receptors on T-helper lymphocytes.
8. The virus then enters the target cell by fusing directly with host cell membrane.
9. A double stranded DNA (provirus) is formed from viral RNA utilizing the enzyme reverse transcriptase.
10. The provirus integrates into host cell's DNA.
11. The provirus remains sequestered from host immune defences within the CD4 lymphocytes.
12. It may be activated to transcribe mRNA and genomic RNA, leading to protein synthesis, assembly, and new virion formation.
13. Mitogens, antigens, and cytokines such as tumor necrosis factor alpha (TNF-α), IL-6, and granulocyte-macrophage colony stimulating factor (GM-CSF) may induce the active replication of the latent vims.
14. New viruses bud out from the host cell membrane.
15. The newly formed gp 120 spikes bind to surrounding CD4 molecules on adjacent cells, and tear holes in their membrane. The punctured cells swell and die.
16. Syncytium may form when the gp 120 of infected cell binds to CD4 receptor on healthy cells. Thus many cells fuse to form the giant cell "Syncytium". Syncytia die soon after formation.

The manifestations of AIDS are secondary to the defects in the cell-mediated immunity. The main cause of the immune defect in AIDS is a quantitative and qualitative deficiency of the helper/inducer lymphocytes. The CD4 (helper/inducer) lymphocyte has been described as the conductor of immunological orchestra and influences the function of many other celts in the immune system. The immune abnormalities in AIDS are summarized in Table 22.5.

Table 22.5: Immunological abnormalities in AIDS

I. Defect in T-cells
   (a) Lymphopenia
   (b) Reduced CD4 (helper/inducer) lymphocytes
   (c) Interference of the interaction between CD4 molecule and its natural ligand, major histocompatibility (MHC) class II molecule by HIV protein
   (d) Elevation in the number of CD8 (suppressor/cytotoxic) lymphocytes
   (e) Inversion of the normal CD4: CD8 ratio
   (f) Abnormalities in the function of CD8 lymphocytes
   (g) Decreased or absent delayed hypersensitivity to both recall and new antigens
   (h) Decreased *in vitro* lymphocyte proliferation responses to:
      1. Mitogens
      2. Antigens
      3. Alloantigens

II. Defects in B-cells
   (a) Abnormality of B-lymphocyte function and immunoregulation
   (b) Polyclonal activation of B-cells
   (c) Hypergammaglobulinemia
   (d) Circulating Immune Complexes (CIC)
   (e) Defective de novo antibody response to new antigens.

III. Natural killer cells
   (a) Defective natural killer (NK) cell function that can be restored by *in vitro* addition of interleukin-2.

IV. Monocytes
   (a) Functional abnormalities
      1. Defective chemotaxis
      2. Defective cytotoxic function
      3. Defective presentation of antigens to T-cells
      4. Defective secretion of Interleukin-1

V. Others
   (a) Circulating acid-labile alpha interferon
   (b) Non-specific anti-lymphocyte antibodies
   (c) Elevated alpha-1 thymosin levels
   (d) Elevated beta-2 microglobulin levels
   (e) Decreased serum thymulin levels
   (f) Increasing soluble interleukin-2 receptor level

AIDS selectively affects "at risk" individuals namely:

- Homosexuals
- Drug abusers
- Hemo-philiacs
- Blood transfusion recipients
- Sexual partners of AIDS patients
- Offsprings of AIDS patients

AIDS can be transmitted through the following routes:

- Infected body secretions: Semen, blood, vaginal secretions
- Infected needles in intravenous drugs users
- Factor VIII concentrates prepared from pooled plasma
- Other blood transfusion products
- Transplacental/perinatal/postnatal

Incubation period usually is less than 5 years with a mean of 27.5 months.

Table 22.6: HIV disease: CDC classification

Group I :	Primary HIV Infection			
Group II :	Asymptomatic Infection			
Group III :	Generalized lymphadenopathy			
Group IV :	AIDS			
	Subgroup A :	Constitutional disease		
	Subgroup B :	Neurologic disease		
	Subgroup C :	Secondary infectious disease		
		C-1 :	Specified Infections from surveillance definition of AIDS	
			Pneumocystis carinii pneumonia	
			Cryptosporidiosis, chronic	
			Isosporiasis	
			Strongyloidiasis, extraintestinal	
			Candidiasis of esophagus, trachea or bronchi	
			Cryptococcosis, extrapulmonary	
			Histoplasmosis, disseminated	
			Mycobacterium avium-intercellulare or	
			M. kansasii disseminated	
			Cytomegalovirus infection	
			Herpes simplex, chronic mucocutaneous or disseminated	
			Progressive multifocal leukoencephalopathy	
		C-2 :	Other specified infectious diseases	
			Hairy leukoplakia, oral	
			Multidermatomal herpes zoster	
			Recurrent *Salmonella* bacteremia	
			Nocardiosis	
			M. tuberculosis, extrapulmonary	
			Oral Thrush	
	Subgroup D :	Secondary Cancers		
		Kaposi's sarcoma		
		Non-Hodgkins lymphoma		
		Primary lymphoma of the brain		
	Subgroup E :	Others		

CLINICAL FEATURES

HIV infection is conceived to form a spectrum of clinical manifestations associated with immune dysfunction. This spectrum reflects the progression of HIV infection from the appearance of initial signs and symptoms through a long asymptomatic period with or without development of generalized lymphadenopathy to the development of AIDS . The CDC classification of HIV disease is shown in Table 22.6.

Another classification for adult patients with HIV infection is the Walter Reed's (WR) classification. The patient is thoroughly examined for the clinical manifestation of HIV disease, screened for antibodies to HIV using ELISA, the positive results of which are then confirmed by Western blot, a T-helper cell count is obtained, and also anergy screen is done by skin testing with mumps, tetanus, trichophyton, and monilial antigens. Patient is then graded on the basis of these results.

WR0 : antibody negative patient with sexual contact with patient with HIV infection.
WR1 : positive culture for, or 2 positive Western blots of HIV.
WR2 : 2 positive Western blots and chronic lymphadenopathy
WR3 : 2 positive Western blots and persistent T-helper cell depletion.

WR4 : 2 positive Western blots, persistent T-helper cell depletion and partial defects in delayed hypersensitivity (DH).

WR5 : 2 positive Western blots, T-helper cell depletion, and either a clinical thrush or persistent anergy.

WR6 : 2 positive Western blots and an opportunistic infection.

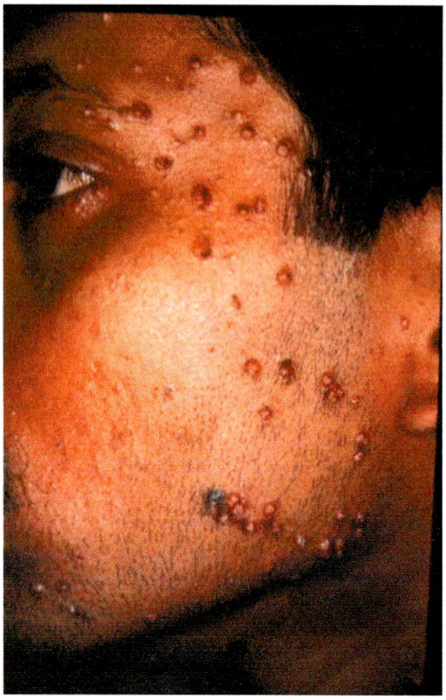

Fig. 22.2: D_1 Molluscum contagiosum

The majority of individuals do not experience signs and symptom at the time of primary infection. However, some may develop fever, rigors, athralgias, myalgias, diarrhea, and aseptic meningitis 3 to 6 weeks after infection. These constitutional symptoms may last for 2 to 3 weeks and then resolve spontaneously.

The acute illness of primary infection is followed by a period of asymptomatic infection. Eight to ten years may elapse before the development of full blown AIDS. 80 to 90 percent of the infected patients will reveal immunologic deterioration within 3 years of infection, though the clinical symptoms may be lacking. Approximately 75 percent of infected individuals develop some symptoms within the first 7 years.

Certain individuals develop persistent generalized lymphadenopathy (PGL) characterized by enlargement of lymph nodes greater than 1 cm at two or more extrainguinal sites that persist for more than 3 months, in the absence of concurrent illness or condition other than HIV infection to explain the lymphadenopathy.

After the varying interval of 8 to 10 years, the patients develop full blown AIDS. This may be heralded by:

- Fever persisting for more than 1 month
- Involuntary weight loss greater than 10 percent
- Diarrhea persisting for more than 1 month.

The constitutional symptoms may be followed by secondary infections. The microorganisms that rarely cause disease in immunologically normal people may be responsible for opportunistic infections in AIDS. The most common sites for such secondary infection are the lungs, pharynx, esophagus, small intestine, bowel, colon, bloodstream, central nervous system, and skin. Systemic manifestations may differ from organ to organ.

Cutaneous Manifestations

The skin is commonly affected in patients with human immunodeficiency virus (HIV) infection. Viral, bacterial, fungal, protozoal infections and ectoparasitic infestation may affect the skin primarily or secondarily. The clinical features are cardinal. However, the lesion bends to be severe, persistent, and resistant to treatment. Unusual inflammatory dermatoses and neoplasms may develop (Table 22.7).

Kaposi's Sarcoma

It presents with one or more asymptomatic faint pink to red macules, papules, blue purple plaques or nodules of variable size. These lesions differ from classic Kaposi sarcoma by their generally

Table 22.7: Cutaneous manifestations of AIDS

I.	Neoplastic	VIII.	Protozoal
	Kaposi's sarcoma		Amebiasis cutis
	B-cell lymphoma	IX.	Arthropod infestation
	Squamous cell carcinoma		Scabies (Norwegian)
	Basal cell carcinoma	X.	Vascular lesions
II.	Viral infections		Vasculitis
	Herpes zoster		Telangiectasia
	Herpes simplex		Thrombocytopenic purpura
	Molluscum contagiosum (Fig. 22.2)		Pseudothrombophlebitis, hyperalgesic
	Warts	XI.	Papulosquamous
	Condylomata acuminata		Psoriasis
	Cytomegalovirus infection		Seborrheic dermatitis
	Oral hairy leukoplakia	XII.	Oral
III.	Bacterial infection		Apthous ulcers
	Pyodermas, some due to commensal floras		Gingivitis
	Ulcers *(Pseudomonas* and polymicrobial)	XIII.	Hairs
IV.	Spirochaetal		Premature graying
	Atypical/malignant syphilis		Telogen effluvium
V.	Mycobacterial	XIV.	Nails
	Disseminated cutaneous tuberculosis		Color changes
	Atypical mycobacterial infection		Deformities
VI.	Candidiasis	XV.	Miscellaneous
VII.	Fungal infection		Exanthems
	Dermatophytosis		Xerosis
	Pityriasis versicolor		Ichthyosis
	Cryptococcosis		Pruritus
	Histoplasmosis		

smaller size, tendency to elongate along lines of cutaneous cleavage, and their lack of propensity to involve primarily the lower extremities. Some patients have persistent generalized lymphadenopathy before the onset of the cutaneous lesions. Kaposi's sarcoma in AIDS patients also has a high incidence of visceral involvement. Chemotherapeutic regimens comprising donorubicin, bleomycin vinblastine have been largely ineffective and have shown complete response is only 15 percent of AIDS Kaposi's sarcoma (Table 22.8).

DIAGNOSIS

The diagnosis of HIV infection is accomplished by performing a battery of diagnostic tests. The most widely used is a test for HIV antibody employing enzyme linked immunosorbent assay (ELISA). This sensitive test is useful in screening large number of individuals for HIV infection. More than 95 percent of HIV-infected persons will be identified as positive by ELISA within 3 months of infection. Its major disadvantage is the relatively high incidence of false positive reactions. The rate of false positive reactions with first generation ELISA, which employs lysates from the HIV infected cells as a source of antigen, has been reduced with second generation ELISA, that utilizes recombinant DNA protein as a source of antigen. All positive ELISA tests should be repeated and if the repeat test is also positive, it should be confirmed by a more specific test for the antibody.

The more specific antibody test used to confirm results of ELISA is the Western blot. The Western blot assay, expensive and more specific, is a confirmatory test and rules out false positive results. It

Table 22.8: Differences between classical and epidemic (AIDS) Kaposi's sarcoma

	Classical Kaposi's sarcoma	*Epidemic (AIDS) Kaposi's sarcoma*
Risk group	Affects older individuals usually in 6th or 7th decade	Young homosexual men. May also affect intravenous drug users, hemophiliacs.
Lesions	Bluish red or dark brown plaques or nodules	Bluish red or dark brown papules, plaques or nodules
Size	Large	Small
Number	A few	Multifocal and widespread oval, arranged along lines of body cleavage in mirror image distribution
Location	Lower extremities	Trunk, head, and neck
Mucosal involvement	May or may not be present	Adjacent mucosae frequently involved
Lymph node involvement	Involved in only 10 percent cases	Frequent. More than half of the patients have generalized lymphadenopathy at presentation. KS may involve lymph nodes in the absence of skin and mucosal lesion.
Visceral involvement	Uncommon	May involve all viscera except brain
Histopathology	1. Vascular formation 2. Spindle cell formation containing vascular slits 3. Inflammatory reaction resembling 'Granulation tissue'	1. Dissection of collagen 2. Lymphatic vessel like space 3. Angiomatoid proliferation 4. Premonitory sign 5. Spindle cell proliferation
Treatment	Surgical excision, radiation therapy, combination chemotherapy	Immune rescue more effective than chemotherapy 1. Human gamma interferon 2. Combination chemotherapy

identifies antibodies against specific viral proteins such as p24, the major HIV protein, and gp 41, gp120, and gp160, the transmembrane and viral envelope proteins. The radioimmunoprecipitation assay (RIPA) is used in research laboratories to further clarify atypical or indeterminate Western blot results. However, it presents difficulty in standardization, sensitivity, and specificity.

The above tests rely upon the detection of antibodies to HIV. However, the antibodies do not appear for weeks or months, following infection. 95 percent of infected individuals develop antibodies within 5 months of infection. Occasionally, the antibody response may be delayed for 3 to 4 years. Under these circumstances, demonstration of the virus is necessary for the diagnosis of HIV infection. The test devised includes detection of p24 antigen, the major core protein of HIV. It is useful for monitoring the efficacy of the therapy. A latex agglutination test has been developed that detects gp 120, the major HIV envelope glycoprotein.

Another highly sensitive test for detecting the virus is the polymerase chain reaction (PCR), which selectively amplifies viral genome allowing detection of HIV DNA present at very low levels in infected cells.

Viral culture remains the ultimate for diagnosing the HIV infection. The test procedure, however, is technically difficult, and expensive.

A brief summary of the diagnostic tests for HIV infection is given in Table 22.9.

A summary of the evolution of HIV markers following infection with HIV is given in Table 22.10.

Besides the diagnostic test for AIDS, a battery of other investigation should be performed in AIDS (Table 22.11).

Table 22.9: Diagnostic tests for HIV infection

Tests	*Advantages*	*Disadvantages*	*Status*
1. ELISA			
1st generation	Sensitive	False positive reactions	Screening test
2nd generation	Sensitive Lower incidence of false positive reactions	—	Screening test
2. Western blot	Specific Rules out false positive results of ELISA	Expensive	Diagnostic
3. RIPA	Clarifies atypical or indeterminate Western blots	Not yet standardized	For research
4. Detection of p24 antigen	Useful for monitoring the efficacy of antiviral therapy	p24 may not be detectable during the course of disease in some	Not yet used routinely
5. Latex agglutination test to detect gp 120	Inexpensive, rapid, easy to use	Unstable Unreliable	Not routinely used
6. Polymerase chain reaction (PCR)	Highly sensitive test Detects even non-replicating virus	False positive results can occur	Not well-standardized as yet
7. Viral culture	Most specific test	Technically difficult Expensive	Not for routine use

Table 22.10: Summary of evolution of markers for HIV infection

Stage of infection	*p24 antigen*	*anti-HIV*	*Western blot pattern*
Immediately after infection	$- \rightarrow +$	—	—
Acute illness	$+ \rightarrow -$	$\pm \rightarrow +$	Restricted, often p24 and/or gp 120
Carrier, asymptomatic	–	+	Full pattern
Carrier, with symptomatic PGL	+	+	Loss of anti p24
AIDS	+	+	Absence of anti-p24

Table 22.11: Other tests to be performed in AIDS

1. Hemoglobin concentration
2. Total-and differential leukocyte counts
3. Quantitation of CD4 and CD8 lymphocytes
4. Platelet counts
5. Serologic tests for syphilis
6. β-microglobulin level
7. Hepatitis B and toxoplasma serology
8. Skin tests for tuberculosis and one or more control antigens
9. Skiagram of the chest

TREATMENT

The goals of AIDS therapy are amelioration of symptoms in full blown' AIDS, prevention of disease progression, and/or treatment of Kaposi's sarcoma and opportunistic infections (Figs 22.3 to 22.6). There are four broad approaches to achieve these goals.

1. Anti-retroviral agents
2. Immunorestorative therapy
3. General management
4. Treatment and/or prophylaxis of specific opportunist infections or tumors

Antiretroviral Agents

The different stages in the lifecycle of HIV present a variety of targets for antiviral agents (Table 22.12).

Zidovudine (3'-azido-3'-deoxythymidine, AZT) has been licensed for use in AIDS. It is a potent chain terminator of HIV reverse transcriptase. It suppresses and not eliminates viral replication in circulating lymphocytes. Circulating HIV antigen (p 24) is reduced during treatment. However, it is possible to isolate virus from the cells by cocultivation. If therapy is reduced or discontinued, levels of circulating p 24 antigen rises rapidly. This reinforces the fact that life-long antiretroviral therapy is necessary.

It is well-absorbed from the gastrointestinal tract after oral administration. Its bioavailability is 60 percent and the levels that inhibit HIV replication can be achieved in patients. The half-life of AZT is 1 hour and most of the drug is cleared by hepatic glucuronidation and renal tubular secretion. It also crosses the blood-brain barrier.

It can induce clinical, immunologic, and virologic benefits in patients with severe HIV infection. Patients receiving it have increase in the weight, improved immune function, and decreased incidence of opportunistic infection. The quality of life and survival rate also improves with AZT.

Table 22.12: Sites for antiretroviral activity

Stage in viral replication	*Antiviral agents*
1. Absorption	Soluble CD4: dextran sulphate; sulphated polysaccharides; peptide T; oligopeptides
2. Entry to cell	Membrane stabilizer AL-721
3. Uncoating	—
4. Reverse transcriptase	Inhibitors-Suramin, phosphonoformate HPA-23 Rifabutin Chain terminators- 3'-azido-3' deoxythymidine (zidovudine), 2'-3' dideoxycytidine (dd C), dideoxyinosine (dd 1), fluorothymidine
5. Integration	—
6. Activation	cyclosporin A
7. Transcription	*art* inhibitor-oligonucleotides
8. Translation	Ribarvin *tat* inhibitor pencillamine
9. Post-translation modification	Inhibition of virus-specific protease avorol
10. Glycosylation	Castanospermine deoxynojirimycin
11. Protein kinase C	Xanthote glycryrrhizin
12. Assembly	Interferons Suramin
13. Budding	Hypericine Interferons
14. Syncytial formation	CD4 blocking agents

The principal toxicity of AZT is bone marrow suppression. Anemia and leukopenia are frequently observed. Other side effects include headache, nausea, and vomiting. Some patients develop myalgia. Also vitamin B_{12} deficiency has been reported in AIDS patient receiving AZT.

Other dideoxynucleosids such as 2'3'-deodycytidine (dd C) and 2'3'-dideoxyadnosine (dd A) are under trial as HIV agents.

The details of zidovudine, dd C and dd A are given in Table 22.13.

Immunorestorative Therapy

The immunorestorative therapy relies upon the use of: (i) interferons, and (ii) interleukin-2, (iii) bone marrow transplantation, (iv) infusion of histocompatible lymphocytes.

Interferons are polypeptides classified into interferon-alpha (1FN-α), interferon-beta (IFN-β), and interferon-gamma (IFN-γ), based upon different antigenic, physiochemical, and biological basis. They were initially regarded as antiviral substances, but their antiproliferative, antitumoral, and immunomodulator properties have been established. Their uses in AIDS are summarized in Table 22.14.

Interleukin-2: It is a glycoprotein released from activated helper T cells in response to either antigen presentation macrophages and Langerhan cells or interleukin-1. It promotes proliferation of activated T cells and promote secretion of lymphokines such as gamma interferon (IFN-γ). It also augments the cytotoxicity to natural killer cells (NK) and lymphocyte activated killer cells (LAK).

It is used either in the natural or recombinant form. The natural form is administered as 24,000 to 1 million units/M^2 weekly for 4 weeks. Recombinant interleukin-2 is administered either as 1 million units/kg boiler infusion or as 3000 to 10,000 units/kg/ hr by infusion. The immune reconstitution achieved is only temporary.

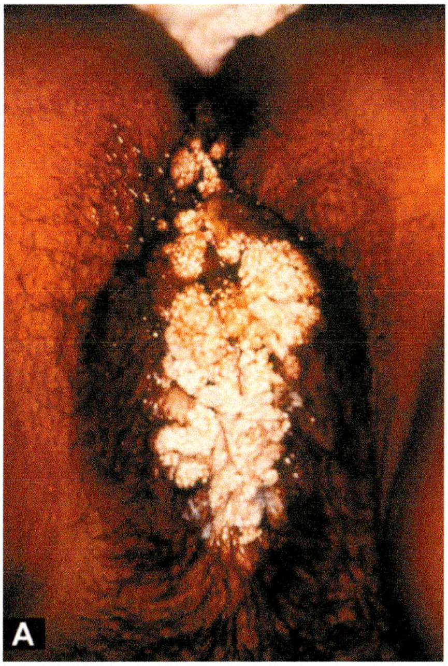

Fig. 22.3A: A_1 Condylomata acuminata (female)

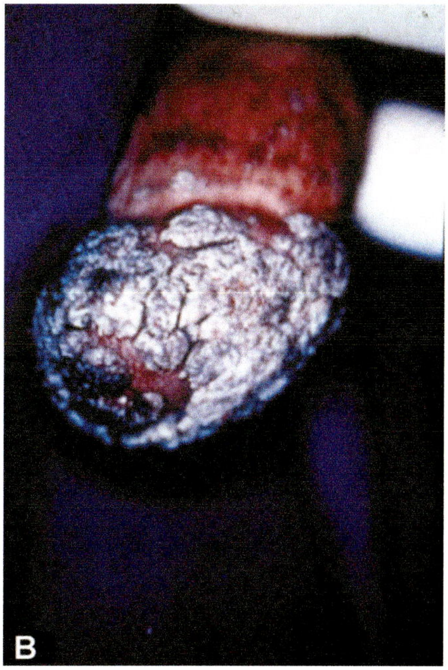

Fig. 22.3B: G_1 Giant condylomata acuminata (male)

Table 22.13: Antiviral agents in the treatment of HIV infection

Anteroviral	*Mode of action*	*Activity*	*Dose*	*Adverse effects*	*Other notes*
Reverse Transcriptase Inhibitors (RTI) a. Nucleoside RTI					
1. Zidovudine (AZT)	Nucleoside analogues are structurally similar to the natural dideoxynucleosides that the HIV reverse transcriptase incorporates into a growing, complementary DNA strand. The nucleoside analogues are incorprated into the growing DNA strand and prevent subsequent elongation	1. Rise in CD4 + count of 50 × 10^{6}/ liter 2. Fall in RNA of about 0.5 log 3. Initiation of AZT monotherapy in asymptomatic patient is associated with a reduced progression of disease 4. AZT < ddI AZT < AZT + ddI AZT < AZT + ddC	**Adults:** 600 mg/day, either as 200 mg every 8 hours of 300 mg every 12 hours **Pediatric:** 180 mg/m^2 every 6 hour	Neutropenia, and anemia; macrocytosis Nausea, headache, and insomnia Myositis and elevation of cretaining phosphokinase, muscle tenderness and wasting	1. AZT is glucuronidated in liver to an inactive metabolite that is excreted by kidneys 2. Probenecid decrease the renal exeretion or inhibits the metabolism of AZT Concomitant administration of these agents may result in flu like symptoms 3. Concomitant administration of AZT with other myelosuppressive agents may increase the toxicity
2. ddC (Zalcitabine)	Nucleoside analogues are structurally similar to the natural dideoxynucleosides that the HIV reverse transcriptase incorporates into a growing, complementary DNA strand. The nucleoside analogues are incorporated into the growing DNA strand and prevent subsequent elongation. Most potent of the antiretroviral nucleoside analogue	AZT + ddC > AZT ddC > ddI Suppression of HIV replication AZT/ddC = AZT/ddI CD4 + cell rise AZT + ddC < AZT + ddI	**Adults:** 0.75 mg every 8 hour	Peripheral neuropathy Burning sensation and pain in the distal extremities Pancreatitis, hepatitis, aphthous ulceration of the mouth and esophagus Rash and stomatitis Anemia, leukopenia, and thrombocytopenia. Fever, malaise, ototoxicity	1. ddC should be taken empty stomach 2. Magnesium and aluminium containing antacids may decrease the bioavailability ddC. Probenecid increases it 3. ddC is eliminated by kidneys and concomitant administration of nephrotoxic drugs may potentially increase the risk of toxicity 4. ddC should be used cautiously in combination with drug that may cause peripheral neuropathy or pancreatitis.
3. ddI (didanosine)	Nucleoside analogues are structurally similar to the natural dideoxynucleosides that the HIV reverse and transcriptase incorporates into a grow ing, complementary DNA strand. The nucleoside analoguesare incorporated into the growing DNA strand areprevent subsequent elongation ddI is a prodrug for the active intracellular metabolite dd ATP	AZT/ddI > AZT (Both AZT naïve AZT-experienced patients)	ddI is available as chewable tablet, and powder for oral solution **Adult:** 200 mg every 12 hour for pts ≥ 60 kg 125 mg every 12 hours for pts ≤ 60 kg	Reversible peripheral neuropathy Pancreatitis, hepatitis Headache, insomnia Uric acid elevation Rash, seizures	ddI is acid labile and is formulated with buffering agents to increase its bioavailability. Concomitant administration of ddI with drugs that require gastric acid for absorption (Ketoconazole, itraconazole) results in decreased bioavailability of these drugs
4. d 4T (stavudine)	Nucleoside analogue are structurally similar to the natural dideoxynucleosides that the HIV reverse transcriptase incorporates into a growing complementary DNA strand. The nucleoside analogues are incorporated into the growing DNA strand and prevent subsequent elongation	1. d 4T > AZT (in AZT experienced patients) d4T is a. better tolerated b. produces greater gains in weight c. results in better life quality 2. d4 T/ddI results in 1 log fall in HIV load in 50% of patients 3. d4T/3TC is well-tolerated and is associated with a rise in CD4 and a fall in HIV load of upto 2 log.	**Adults:** Body weight ≥ 60 kg 40 mg every 12 hours Body weight ≤ 60 kg 30 mg every 12 hours **Pediatric:** 0.125 to 2 mg/kg every 12 hours	Peripheral neuropathy Anemia, neutropenia GIT disturbance and pancreatics Elevated hepatic transaminases	d 4T must be used cautiously in combination with other agents that cause peripheral neuropathy (isoniazid and metronidazole)

Contd.

Contd.

Anteroviral	*Mode of action*	*Activity*	*Dose*	*Adverse effects*	*Other notes*
5. 3 TC (Lamivudine)	Nucleoside analogues are structurally similar to the natural dideoxynucleosides that the HIV reverse transcriptase incorporates into a growing, complementary DNA strand. The nucleoside analogues are incorporated into the growing DNA strand and prevent subsequent elongated	1. 3 TC monotherapy produces a rapid but transient fall in RNA levels 2. Loss of HIV suppression is associated with a rapid development of resistance resulting from a single point mutation at codon 184 of HIV RT 3. AZT/ 3TC combination produces a prolonged and sustained CD4+ elevation 4. In AZT naïve patients, 3TC/AZT produces a sustained Suppression of HIV RNA at 1year and an increase in CD4 + counts of 80 × 10^6/litre 5. AZT/3TC produces a 30-40 × 10^6/litre increase in CD4+ and 0.5 log fall in HIV in AZT treated cases	**Adults:** Body weight $\geq$ 50 kg 150 mg every 12 hour Body weight $\leq$ 50 kg 2 mg/kg body weight every 12 hours	Elevation of serum amylase Pancreatitis peripheral neuropathy	1. 3 TC may be taken without regards to meals 2. 3 TC increase peak serum levels of AZT
b. Non-nucleoside RTI (NNRTI)					
1. Nevirapine	NNRTI are structurally dissimilar to the nucleoside RTIs and bind at distinct sites on the RT enzyme	1. Exerts transient antiretroviral effect that wanes with the development of nevirapine resistance 2. AZT/ddI/navirapine (greater viral load suppression at 8 weeks and more sustained CD4+ rise) 3. AZT naïve, asymptomatic patients treated with AZT/ddI/nevirapine experience an increase in CD 4^+ count of 100 × 10^6/litre and 50% have viral load suppression to fewer than 20 copies/ml 4. Rapid resistance on monotherapy with nevirapine	200 mg orally, once a day, for 14 days followed by 200 mg twice a day	Skin rash fatigue Diarrhea raised liver function tests Headache and depression	1. Nevirapine may be taken without regards to meal 2. Patients may be instructed to report any skin rash while receiving the drug 3. It decrease AZT bioavailability 4. It induces liver enzymes and has the potential to intact with drug metabolized through cytochrome p 450 5. Rifampicin must not be administered commitanfy with nevirapine
2. Delaviridine	NNRTI are structurally dissimilar to the nucleoside RTIs and bind at distinct sites on RT enzyme	AZT/delaviridine = ddI/delaviridine AZT/delaviridine results in a. decrease in viral RNA of 0.5 log b. $CD4^+$ increase of 20-30 × 10^6/litre	400 mg thrice a day	Skin, rash Headache fatigue, GI disturbance elevation in LFT anemia thrombocytopenia and neutropenia	1. Delaviridine should be taken with an acidic beverage 2. It may be taken without regards to marks 3. Patients must be advised to report in case any rash develops 4. Drugs that decrease gastric acidity (antacids, H_2 receptor antagonist decrease delaviridine absorption 5. Concomitant administration of ddI decreases bioavailability of delaviridine 6. It is a cytochrome p-450 3 inhibitors

Contd.

Contd.

Anteroviral	*Mode of action*	*Activity*	*Dose*	*Adverse effects*	*Other notes*
Protease inhibitor					
1. Saquinavir	inhibitors of the HIV Protease are potent agents with differing structures that bind at distinct sites on the HIV protease active sites. They suppress HIV replication by inhibiting proteolysis of viral gag and gag-pol polyproteins, rendering progeny virus non-infectious. Protease inhibitors may reduce the HIV load by upto 1000-fold (3 log) and may produce a sustained increase in the $CD4^+$ cell count	1. At standard doses, squinavir exerts a less potent antiretroviral suppression and has less sustained $CD4^+$ cell response than indinavir and ritonavir, Saquinavir < Indinavir, ritonavir 2. In AZT naïve patients, the combination of saquinavir and AZT produces a. 1 log reduction in HIV load b. 70×10^6/liter rise in $CD4^+$ count	saquinavir is available as 200 mg capsules **Adults:** 600 mg (3 × 200) three times a day **Pediatrics:** Safety of saquinavir in the age group is not established	GI disturbances, elevated liver function test, jaundice, seizures, headache, rash	1. Patients should be instructed to take saquinavir within 2 hr of a full meal and each dose should comprise of 3 200 mg capsules 2. Saquinavir has low bioavailability and extensive first pass metabolism by liver 3. It is metabolized by the hepatic cytochrome p 450 degradation of saquinavir is inhibited by ketoconazole, and the protease inhibitor ritonavir
2. Ritonavir	Inhibitors of the HIV protease are potent agents with differing structures that bind at distinct sites on the HIV protease active site. They suppress HIV-replication by inhibiting proteolysis of viral gag and gag-pol polyproteins, rendering progeny virus non-infectious. Protease inhibitors may reduce the HIV load by upto 1000 fold (3 log) and may produce a sustained increase in the $CD4^+$ cell count	1. As monotherapy, ritonavir potently suppresses viral load (a 1.2-2 log reduction at 2 weeks) accompanied by an average increase in $CD4^+$ count of 200×10^6/liter 2. AZT/ddc/ritonavir combination sustains the above effects for 6 or more months 3. In patients with advanced HIV disease with $CD4^+$ well counts below 100×10^6/liter addition of ritonavir to a stable regimen of nucleoside analogue therapy, results in modest effects a. 0.6 log viral load suppression b. $40\text{-}50 \times 10^6$/liter increase in $CD4^+$ counts Theses effects markedly reduce disease progression and the mortality rate	600 mg, twice a day with meals	Nausea, diarrhoea, headache, dizziness circumoral paresthesia vasodilatation, raised hepatic enzymes	1. Ritonavir should be taken with food 2. Ritonavir capsules and solution should be refrigerated 3. Caution should be exercised in prescribing ritonavir in patients with hepatic dysfunction
3. Indinavir	Inhibitors of the HIV protease are potent agents with differing structures that bind at distinct sites on the HIV protease active site. They suppress HIV-replication by inhibiting proteolysis of viral gag and gag-pol polyproteins, rendering progeny virus non-infectious. Protease inhibitors may reduce the HIV load by upto 1000 fold (3 log) and may produce a sustained increase in the CD4 cell count	1. Indinavir reduces viral load by 1.5 log at 6 months in previously untreated patients 2. Same patients on indinavir monotherapy sustain increase of 100×10^6/l $CD4^+$ cells for more than 1 year 3. AZT/indinavir combination therapy shows more marked viral load suppression (1.0-2.6 log), with an average rise in CD4+ count of 100×10^6/liter	**Adults:** 800 mg every 8 hours, taken with water, before or 2 hours after a meal	Nephrolithiasis Asymptomatic indirect hyperbilirubinemia	1. Patients should be instructed to drink plenty of water to minimize the possibility of nephrolithiasis

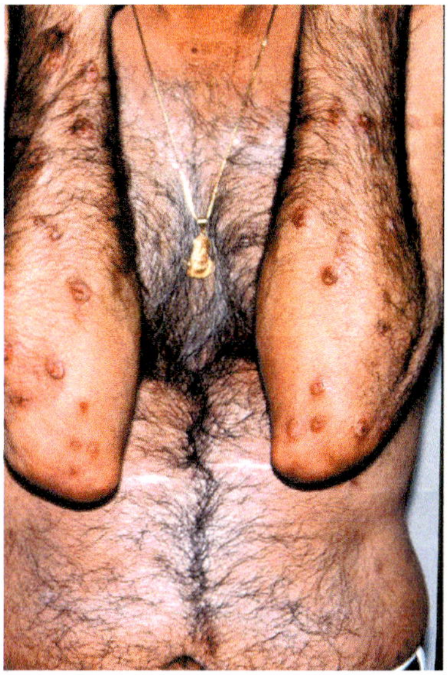

Fig. 22.4: C_1 Syphilis ropial psoriasis

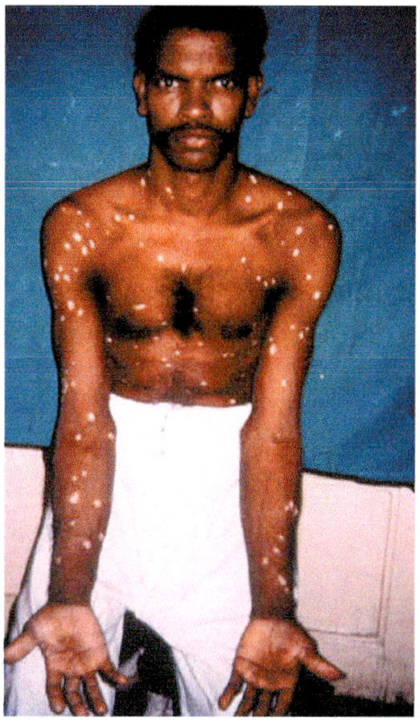

Fig. 22.5: F_1 Prurigo nodularis

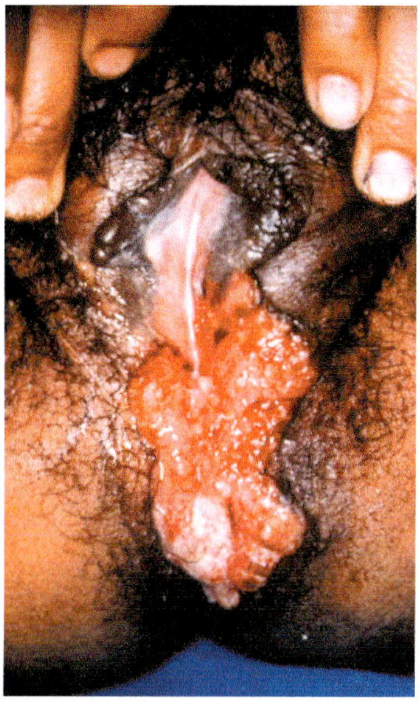

Fig. 22.6: B_1 Donovanosis hypotrophy with SCC

Table 22.14: Interferons in AIDS

Interferons	*Doses*	*Effects*
Alpha-2 interferon	15 million unit/M^2 i/v Or 1 million units/M^2 S/C for 5 days, alternate week for 4 cycles	(1) Augments NK activity (2) Useful in Kaposi's sarcoma
Gamma interferon	1-10 million units/M^2 twice a week by i/v infusion	(1) Augments antibody production (2) Increases macrophage tumoricidal activity (3) Augments NK activity

FURTHER READING

1. Berwick D. "We all have AIDS" case for reducing the cost of HIV drugs to zero. BMJ 2002; 324: 214-6.
2. Blocker ME, Levine WC, St Louis ME. HIV prevalence in patients with syphilis, United States. Sex Transm Dis 2000;27:53-9.
3. Czelusta A, Yen-Moore A, van der Straten M, Carrasco D, Tyring SK. An overview of sexually transmitted diseases. Part III. Sexually transmitted diseases in HIV-infected patients. J Am Acad Dermatol 2000;43:409-32.
4. Dowe G, Smikle M, King SD, Baum M, Chout R, Williams Y. Symptomatic and asymptomatic chlamydial non-gonococcal urethritis in Jamaica: the potential for HIV transmission. Int J STD AIDS 2000;11:187-90.
5. Dal Maso L, Serraino D, Franceschi S. Epidemiology of AIDS-related tumours in developed and developing countries. Eur J Cancer 2001;37:1188-201.
6. D' Amelio R, Tuerlings E, Perito O, Biselli R, Natalicchio S, Kingma S. A global review of legislation on HIV/AIDS: the issue of HIV testing. J Acquir Immune Defic Syndr 2001;28:173-9.
7. El-Attar SM, Evans DV. Anal warts, sexually transmitted diseases, and anorectal conditions associated with human immunodeficiency virus. Prim Car 1999;26:81-100.
8. Fowler VG Jr, Maxwell GI, Myers SA, Shea CR, Livengood CN 3rd, Prieto VG, et al. Failure of benzathine penicillin in a case of seronegative secondary syphilis in a patient with acquired immunodeficiency syndrome: case report and review of the literature. Arch Dermatol 2001;137:1374-6.

9. Goldschmidt RH, Dong BJ. Treatment of AIDS and HIV-related conditions: 2001. J Am Board Fam Pract 2001;14:283-309.
10. Helfgott A. TORCH testing in HIV-infected women. Clin Obstet Gynecol 1999;42:149-62.
11. Ippolito G, Galati V, Serraino D, Girardi E. The changing picture of the HIV/AIDS epidemic. Ann NY Acad Sci 2001;946:1-12.
12. Osemene NI, Essien EJ, Fgbunike IG. HIV/AIDS behind bars: an avenue for culturally sensitive interventions. J Nat I Med Assoc 2001;93:481-6.
13. Rauner MS, Brandeau ML. AIDS policy modeling for the 21st century: an overview of key issues. Health Care Manag Sci 2001;4:165-80.
14. Swica Y, Breithart W. Treating pain in patients with AIDS and a history of substance use. West J Med 2002;176: 33-9.
15. Weller IV, Williams IG. ABC of AIDS. Antiretroviral drugs. BMJ 2001;322:1410-2.
16. de Beer I, Coutinho HM, van Wyk PJ, Gaeb E, Rinke de Wit T, van Vugt M. Anonymous HIV workplace surveys as an advocacy tool for affordable private health insurance in Namibia. J Int AIDS Soc 2009;2:7.

Chapter 23

Syndromic (Symptomatic) Approach

INTRODUCTION

Advent of human immunodeficiency virus (HIV) and acquired immunodeficiency syndrome (AIDS) has warranted a major change in eradicatiton and control of sexually transmitted diseases, for sexual intercourse forms one of the major modes of transmission of HIV. Genitoulcerative disease (GUD), in particular and nongonococcal urethritis (NGU), in general, is a risk factor. The precise diagnosis of STD is a dilemma in situation where laboratory component is not readily available for confirming the clinical impression. At that stage, therefore, symptomatic syndromic approach may be ideal for their instant treatment. This option has now been widely approved and acclaimed, and is illustrated through the Flow charts 23.1 to 23.10, encompassing the various manifestations of STD. This approach may facilitate the management of sexually transmitted disease both at under-privileged health care center and district and/or teaching institutions. Furthermore, it is imperative to emphasize that these outlines should be supplemented by measures to prevent the spread of sexually transmitted diseases by adopting the following yardsticks, namely:

- Treatment
- Instructions for medication and follow-up
- Education and counseling comprising:
  - Cure the reservoir of infection.
  - Do not spread STD.
  - Help your sexual partner to get treatment.
  - Come back to make sure that you are cured.
  - Stay cured with condoms.
  - Keep safety but staying with just one sexual partner.
  - Protect yourself against HIV/AIDS.
  - Protect your baby—ask the patient to attend antenatal check-up in the course of pregnancy.
  - Use of condoms.

Flow chart 23.1: Urethral discharge: Syndromic diagnosis, treatment and follow-up

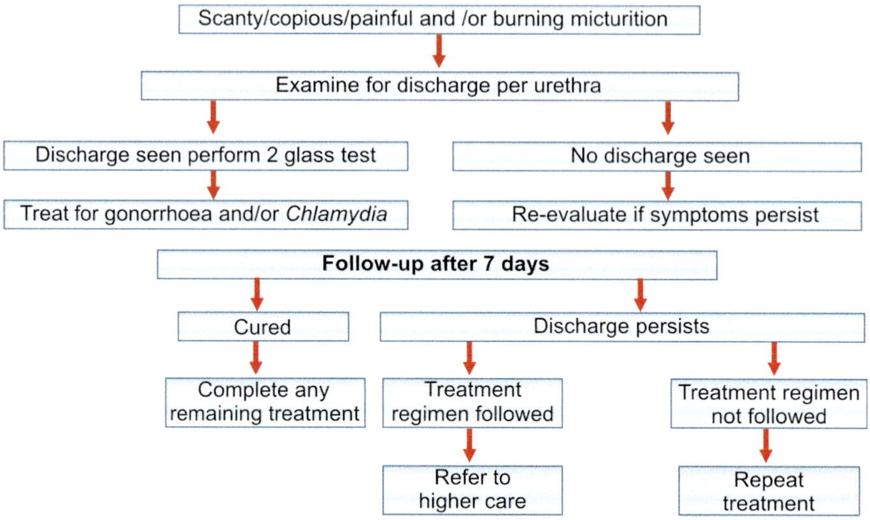

TREATMENT

Gonococcal Urethritis (Gonorrhea)

Institute oral single dose treatment either with

- Ciprofloxacin (Biocip, Cifran, Ciprobid) 500 mg, or
- Cefixime (Cefspan, Taxim-O, Biotax-O) 400 mg, or
- Ceftriaxone (Cemax, Ceftrax, Monocef, Comtrax) 250 to 500 mg by slow intravenous infusion/ intramuscular injection or
- Kanamycin (Kanamac, Kancin) 2 gm by intramuscular injection.

Chlamydia

Institute oral treatment for 7 days' period either with

- Doxycycline (Biodoxi, Doxy-1, Doxt, Microdox-DS) 200 mg a day or
- Minocycline (Cynomycin) 200 mg a day or
- Tetracycline (Hostacycline) 2 gm daily in four divided dosage or
- Erythromycin estolate (Althrocin, Etomin, Eromed-333) 2 gm daily in four divided dosage.

Caution: Ciprofloxacin, tetracycline, doxycycline and minocycline must not be used during pregnancy and/or lactation.

Flow chart 23.2: Urethral discharge: Syndromic and laboratory diagnosis, treatment and follow-up

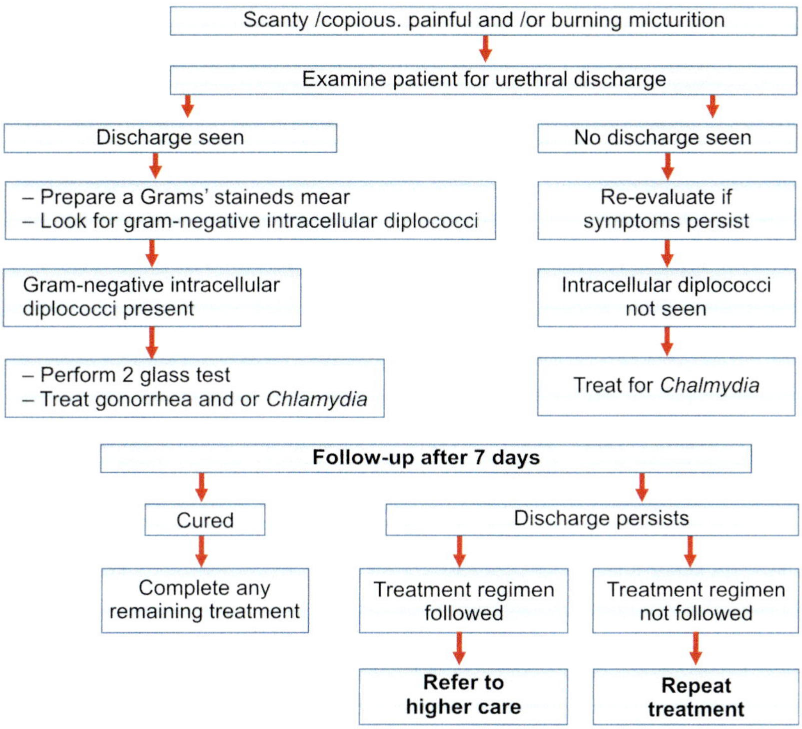

Flow chart 23.3: Inguinal bubo: Uni- or bilateral

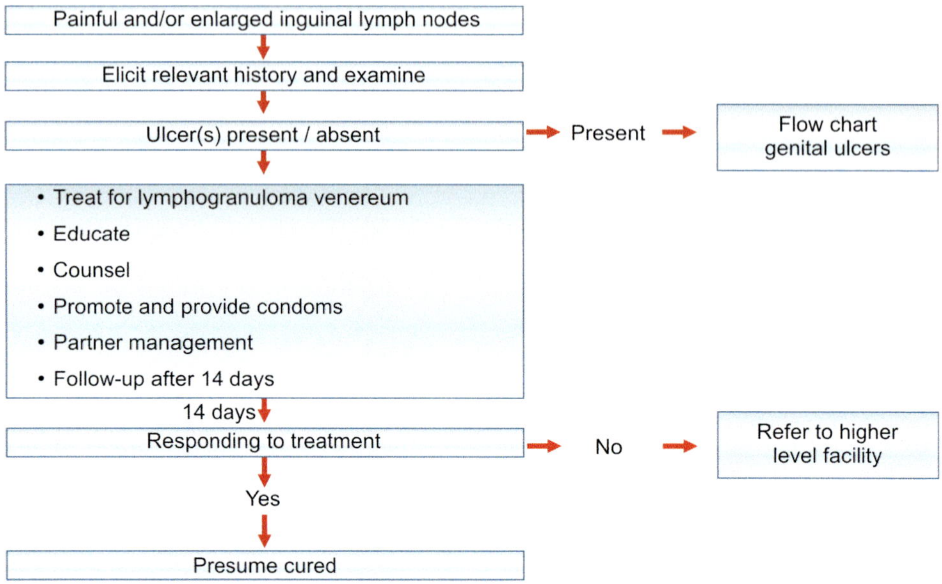

Lymphogranuloma Venereum

Administer either

- Doxycycline (Biodoxi, Doxy 1, Doxt, Microdox-DS) a total of 2.8 grams in divided dosage of 100 mg 2 times a day for 14 days or
- Tetracycline (Hostacycline) a total of 28 grams in the divided dosage of 2 grams daily for a period for 14 days or
- Erythromycin estolate (Althrocin, Etomin, Eromed-333) a total of 28 grams in the divided dosage of 2 grams daily for 14 days. Aspiration of the fluctuant bubo with wide bore neddle may hasten quick recovery.

Flow chart 23.4: Ophthalmia neonatorum (neonatal conjunctivitis)

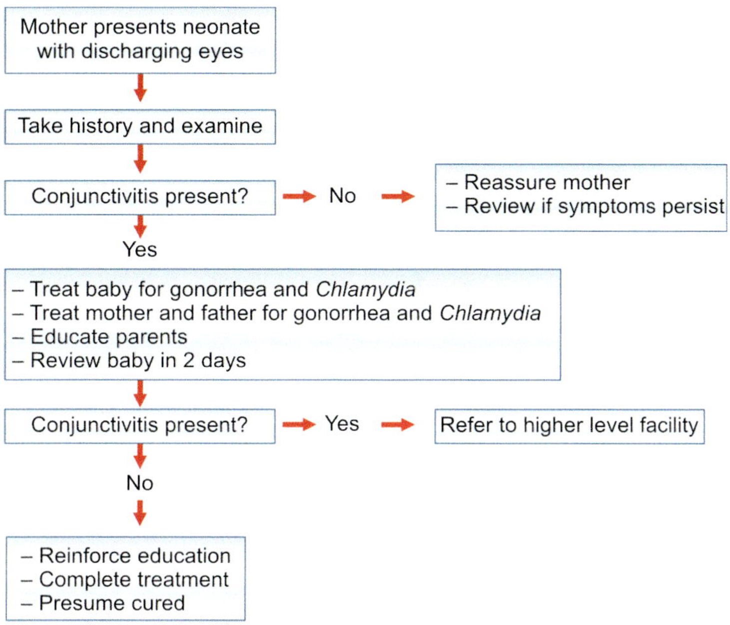

- Ceftriaxone (Cemax, Ceftrax, Monocef, Comtrax) 50 mg/kg body weight by intramuscular injection as a single dose to a maximum of 125 mg.

Alternative Regimen where Ceftriaxone is not Available

- Kanamycin (Kanamac, Kancin) 25 mg/kg body weight by intramuscular injection as a single dose to a maximum of 75 mg or
- Spectinomycin (Trobicin) 25 mg/kg body weight by intramuscular injection as a single dose to a maximum of 75 mg plus
- Erythromycin syrup (Eryc, Althrocin) 50 mg/kg body weight per day orally in 4 divided dosage for 14 days.
- Single dose ceftriaxone, kanamycin and spectinomycin are of proven efficacy.
- The addition of tetracycline eye ointment to these regimens is of no documented benefit.

Flow chart 23.5: Vaginal discharge: Syndromic diagnosis, treatment and follow-up

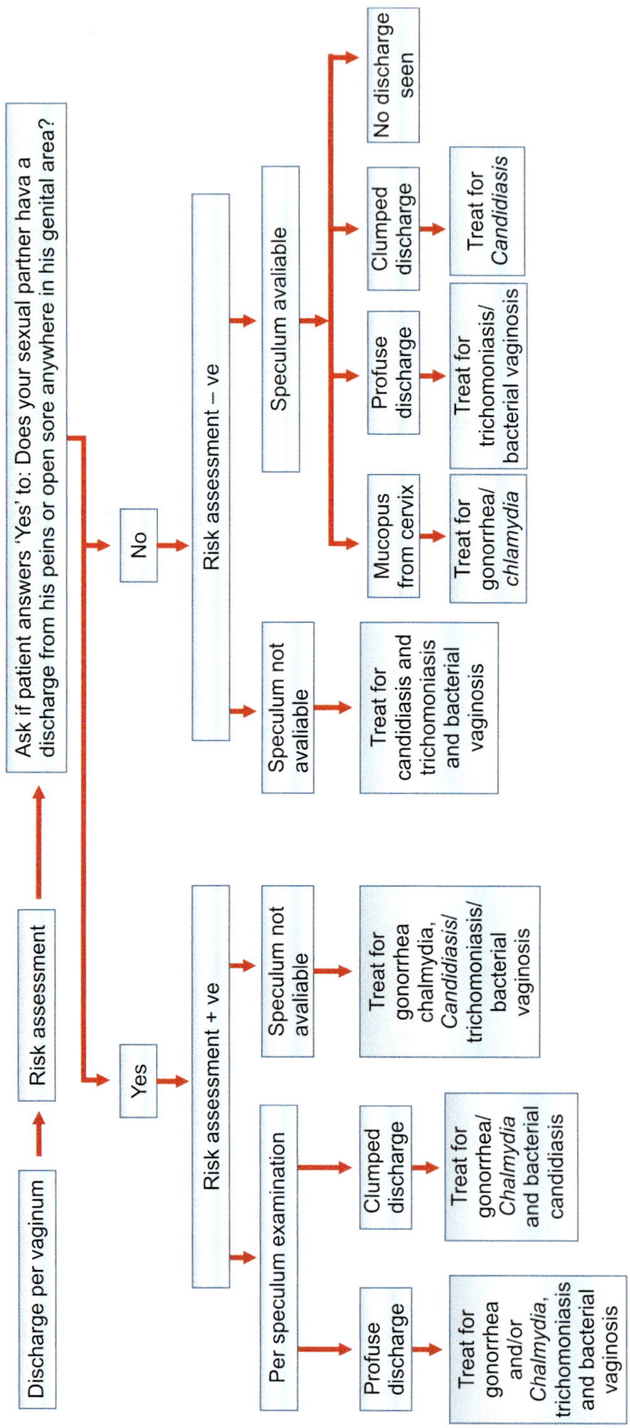

Vaginal Discharge

Should it be gonorrhea and/or *Chlamydia* on per speculum examination, institute oral treatment with

- Ciprofloxacin (Biocip, Cifran, Ciprobid) 500 mg in a single dosage supplemented either by
- Doxycycline (Biodoxi, Doxy 1, Doxt, Microdox-DS) 100 mg 2 times a day up to 1.4 gm in 7 days or
- Minocycline (Cynomycin) 100 mg 2 times a day up to 1.4 gm in 7 days or
- Cerftriaxone (Cemax, Ceftrax, Monocef, Comtrax) 250 to 500 mg by slow intravenous

Preceding Drugs

Preceding drugs are to be avoided in pregnancy and should instead be replaced either by

- Azithromycin (Azithral) 500 mg in a single dose by slow intravenous infusion/intramuscular injection or
- Erythromycin estolate (Althrocin, Etomin, Eromed-333) 500 mg 4 times a day upto 20 to 30 gm for 10 to 15 days
- Metroniazole (Aldezol, Flagyl, Metrogyl) 400 mg 3 times a day or a total of 8.4 gm in equal divided dosage for 7 days period along
- Clotrimazole (Canesten, Candid) 200 mg once a day for 3 days or
- Clotrimazole (Candid, Canesten) 500 mg intravaginally only once a day or
- Fluconazole (Forcan, Fluzon) 150 mg in a single oral dose.

Flow chart 23.6: Vaginal discharge: Syndromic and laboratory diagnosis, treatment and follow-up

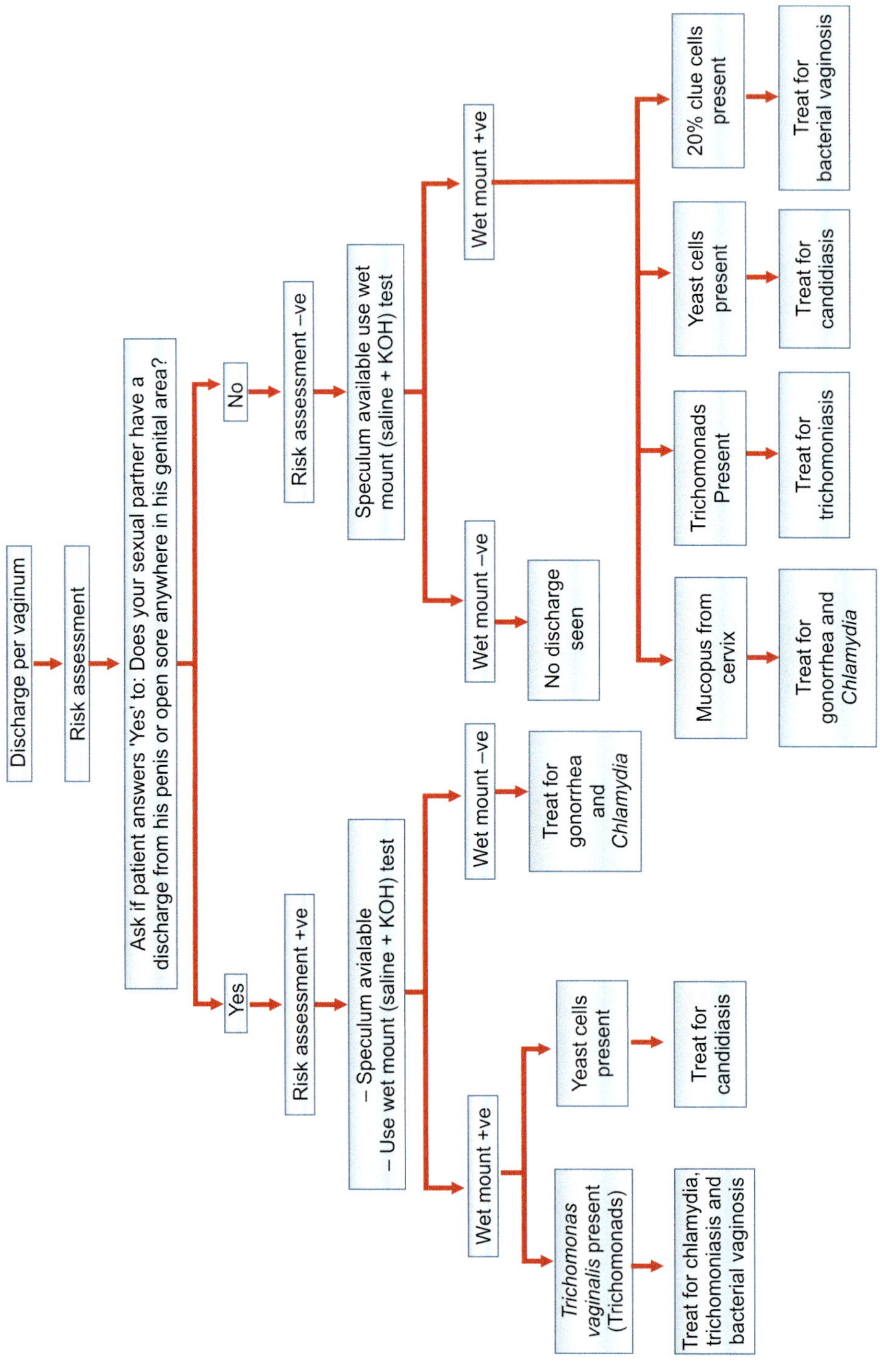

Flow chart 23.7: Genital ulcer: Syndromic diagnosis, treatment and follow-up

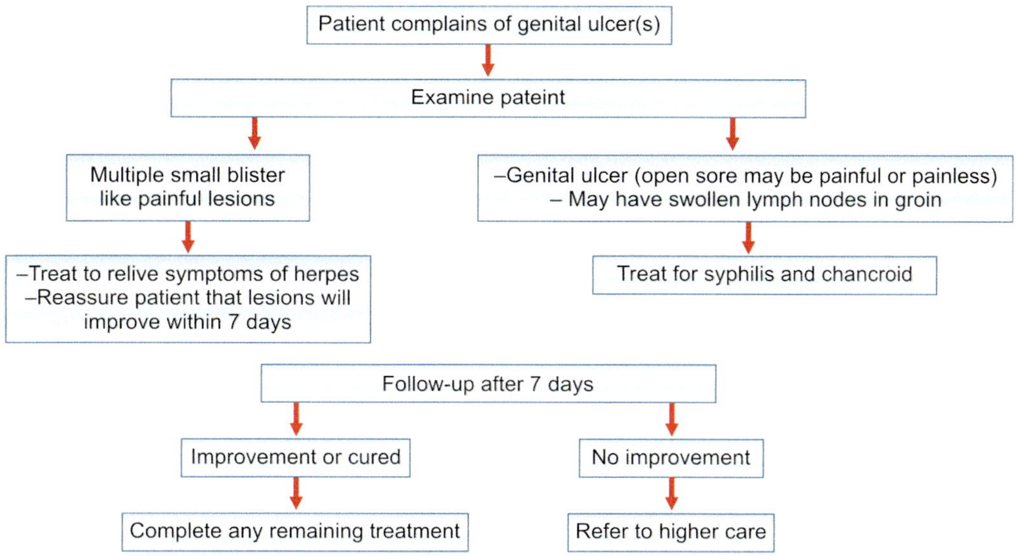

Syphilis, Chancroid and Herpes Progenitalis

Syphilis, chancroid and herpes progenitalis are the major genitoulcerative diseases. Treatment guidlines for the preceding diseases are:

Syphilis: It is treated either by administering

- Benzathine penicillin (Penidure-LA) 2.4 milion units given intramuscular in 2 equal divided dosage of 1.2 million units in each buttock or
- Doxycycline (Biodoxi, Doxy-1, Doxt, Microdox-DR) minocyline (Cynomycin) 100 mg 2 times a day upto a total dose of 2 to 3 gm in 10-15 days or
- Tetracycline (Hostacycline) 500 mg 4 times a day upto 30-40 gm in 10-15 days.
- Erythromycin estolate (Althrocin, Etomin, Eromed-333) 500 mg up to 2-3 gm a day in 10-15 days.

Chancroid: It is treated by oral administration of

- Ciprofloxacin (Cifran, Microflox, Quintor) 500 mg orally in a single dose or
- Trimethroprim 80 mg/sulphamethoxazole 400 mg/(Otrim, Septran) 2 tabs 2 times a day for 7 days or
- Trimethroprim 160 mg/sulphamethoxazole 800 mg (Bactrim, Otrim) 1 tab a day for 7 days or
- Ceftriazone (Ceftrax, Comtrax, Cemax) 1 gm intravenous in a single dose.

Herpes progenitalis: It is treated by oral administeration of

- Acyclovir (Zovirax, Herpex, Herperax) 200 mg 5 times a day for 7 days (first episode)
- Recurrent episode are treated in a similar ways for 5 days.

Caution: Ciprofloxacin, tetracycline, doxycycline and minocycline must not be used during pregnancy and lactation.

Flow chart 23.8: Genital ulcer: Syndromic and laboratory diagnosis, treatment and follow-up

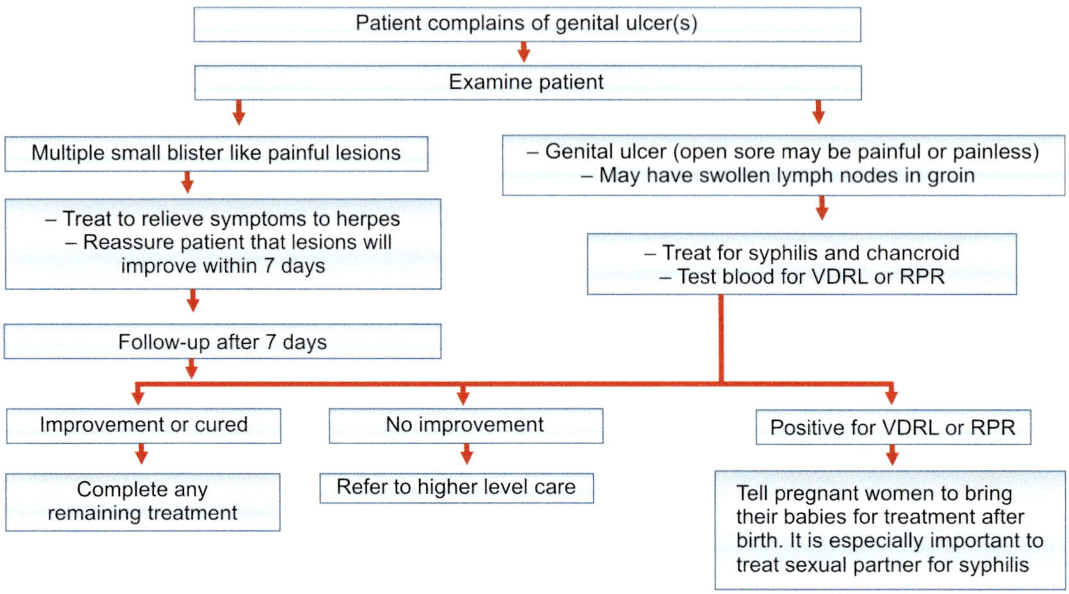

Flow chart 23.9: Sexually transmitted diseases: Scrotal swelling

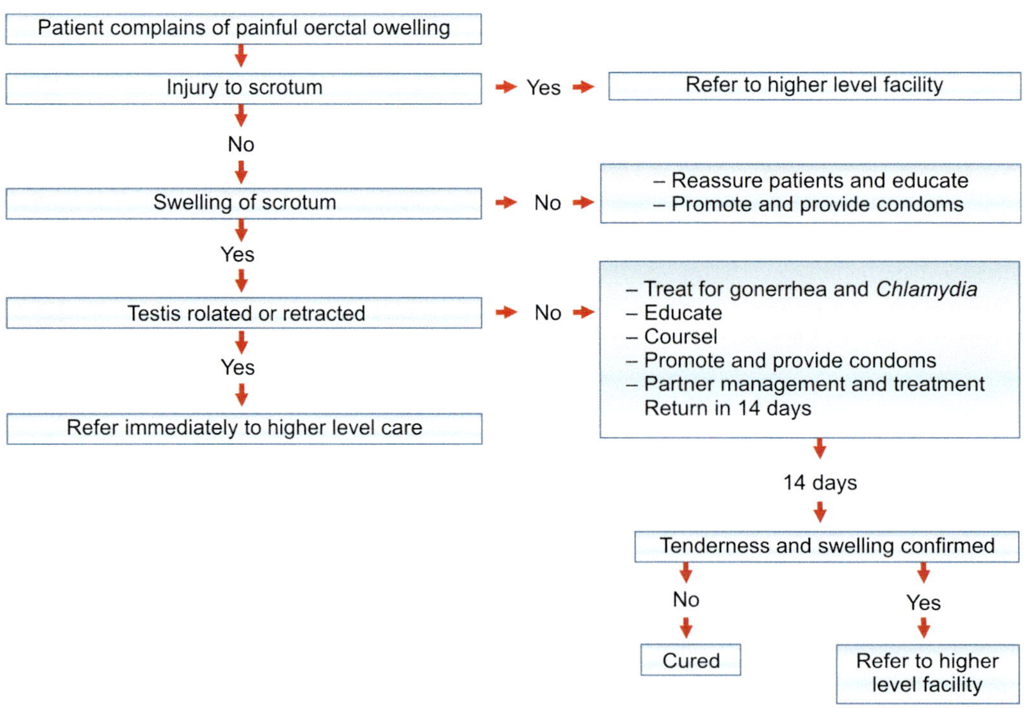

- Ciprofloxacin (Cifran, Microflox, Quintor) 500 mg as a single oral dose (make sure that the patient swallows the tablets under supervision)

Alternative Regimen

- Ceftriaxone (Cemax, Ceftrax, Monocef, Comtrax) 250 mg intramuscular as a single dose or
- Cefixime (Cefspan, Taxim-O, Biotax-O) 400 mg in a single oral dose or
- Kanamycin (Kanamac, Kancin) 2 g intramuscular as a single dose. Recommended regimen for Chlamydia

Urethritis

- Doxycycline (Biodoxi, Doxy 1, Doxt, Microdox-DS) 100 mg orally 2 times a day for 10 days (make sure that the patient receives 20 tablets or capsules with instructions to take one tablet in the morning and one in the evening)

Alternative Regimen

- Tetracycline (Hostacycline) 500 mg orally 4 times a day for 10 days or
- Erythromycin estolate (Althrocin, Etomin, Eromed-333) 500 mg orally 4 times a day for 10 days (equivalent doses of other sulfonamides (triple sulfa) may also be used.)

This is a painful condition and supportive therapy with:

- Bed-rest
- Scrotal elevation with a scrotal support and analgesic is essential part of management
- Advise the patient to take all his tablets and inform him about the mode of transmission of STD and the possible complications of infection and, in particular, epididymo-orchitis.

Flow chart 23.10: Lower abdominal pain in women: Syndromic diagnosis, treatment and follow-up

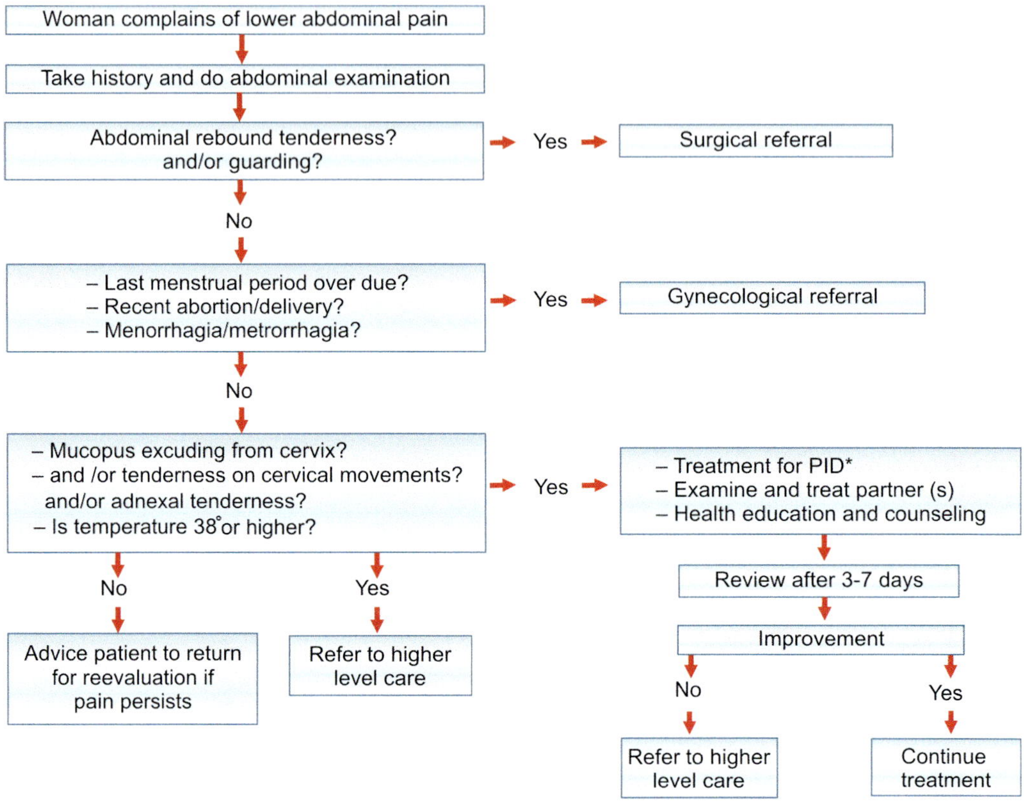

Treatment for Pelvic Inflammatory Disease (PID)

(*N. gonorrhoea* + *C. tricomatis* + anaerobic infection) use this regimen only if patient is well enough to take food and liquid, walk unassisted, take her medication, and return for follow-up. Otherwise, refer to higher level care.

Single Dose Treatment for Gonorrhea

- Ciprofloxacin (Cifran, Ciprobid) 500 mg, orally as a single dose, or
- Ceftriaxone (Cemax, Ceftrax, Monocef, Comtrax) 250 mg to 1 g by slow intravenous infusion/ intramuscular injection as a single dose, or
- Cefixime (Cefspan, Taxim-O, Biotax-O) 400 mg orally as a single dose, or
- Kanamycin (Kanamac, Kancin) 2 gm by intramuscular injection as a single dose.

Alternative Treatment, if Single Dose Treatment is not Available

- Trimethoprim 80 mg/sulfamethoxazole 400 mg (Bactrim, Ciplin, cotrimoxazole) 10 tablets stat daily for 3 days, and then two tablets orally, 2 times a day.

Plus Treatment for Chlamydia tricomatis

- Doxycycline (Biodoxi, Doxy 1, Doxt, Microdox-DS) 100 mg orally 2 times daily for 14 days or
- Tetracycline 500 mg (Hostacycline) orally 4 times daily for 14 days.

Plus Treatment for Anaerobic Infection

- Metronidazole 400 mg (Aldezol, Flagyl, Metrogyl) 2 times daily for 14 days (avoid in 1st trimester of pregnancy, also avoid alcohol)

FURTHER READING

1. Adler MW. Syndromic management of genital ulcer disease. Genitourin Med 1995;71:416.
2. Anonymous. Sexually transmitted diseases treatment guidelines 2002. Centers for Disease Control and Prevention. MMWR Recomm Rep 2002;51:1-78.
3. Htun Y, Morse SA, Dangor Y, Fehler G, Radebe F, Trees DL, et al. Comparison of clinically directed, disease specific, and syndromic protocols for the management of genital ulcer disease in Lesotho. Sex Transm Infect 1998;74:S23-8.
4. Pettifor A, Walsh J, Wilkins V, Raghunathan P. How effective is syndromic management of STDs?: a review of current studies. Sex Transm Dis 2000;27:371-85.
5. Van Dam CJ, Becker KM, Ndowa F, Islam MQ. Syndromic approach to STD case management: where do we go from here? Sex Transm Infect 1998;74:S175-8.

Chapter 24

Prevention and Control of Sexually Transmitted Diseases

INTRODUCTION

In order to outline and understand the prevention and control of sexually transmitted diseases, it is imperative to review the factor(s) responsible for their persistence and perpetual spread. It is, therefore, essential to read the present text in conjunction with that of epidemiology of venereal diseases (Chapter 2). It is paradoxical that in spite of sufficient technical knowledge on how to diagnose and treat, these are the only group of diseases that are on the increase. Most other communicable diseases have been brought either undercontrol or completely eradicated in most parts of the world. It is attributed to a variety of factors comprising poor health information inaccurate or inadequate knowledge of the diseases amongst the general public, administrators, politicians and above all, doctors.

Their effective prevention and control, therefore, need be built around organizing a network of venereal disease clinics, where facilities for early diagnosis, contact tracing, early treatment and follow-up are provided. In addition participation of the administrators, politicians, general practitioners, and health education of the lay public is vital.

ORGANIZATION OF STD SERVICES

It consists of establishing exclusive clinics at different levels. The clinics may be named as sexually transmitted disease (STD) clinics, thus minimising the social stigma attached to VD and attracting a larger number of patients. The clinics should consist of Urban STD centers having ramifications (sub-centers) in the rural areas, regional STD centres, reference laboratory and a central controlling authority for the purpose of administration (Fig. 24.1). The controlling authority should preferably be at the center, dispensing the dual control of the state and the center existing in most countries at present, thus ensuring greater coordination. Active support and collaboration of the general practitioners, consultants, and general hospitals should also be solicited. These centers should have adequate space, doctors, nurses and paramedical workers, well-trained in handling sexually transmitted diseases. The services can be made more effective, should the doctors with postgraduate qualifications head the clinics.

DIAGNOSTIC FACILITIES

Adequate laboratory facilities for confirming the clinical diagnosis is the mainstay in the control of STD. These facilities should essentially comprise smears (Gram's and Leishman's stain), wet preparations (dark-ground, saline and KOH), culture and sensitivity (instant and referral cultures),

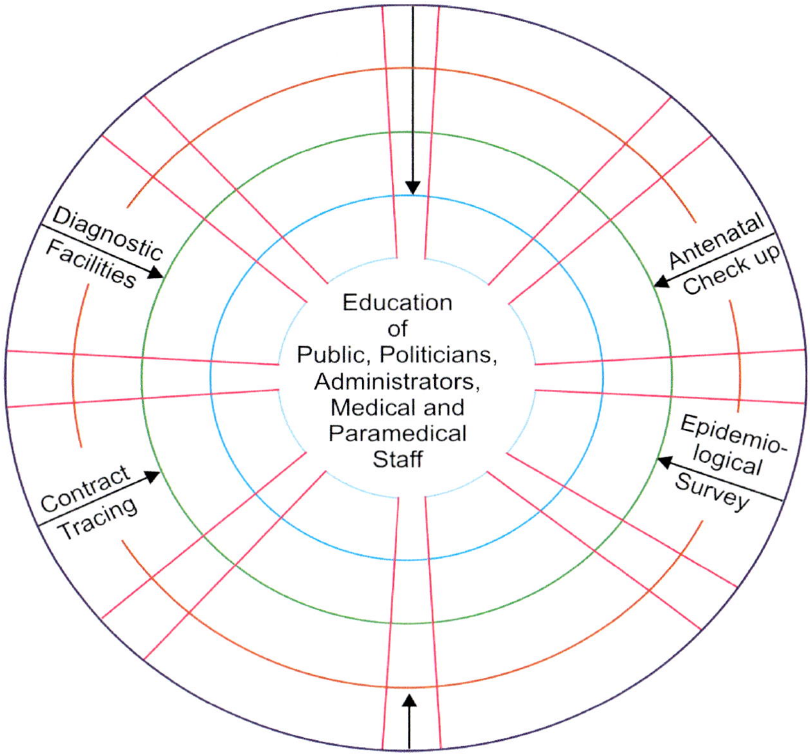

Fig. 24.1: Planning and organization of STD services

standard tests for syphilis and ELISA for HIV antibodies. The latter two may preferably be carried out at the clinic or sent to the regional reference laboratory. Facilities may be made available at the reference laboratory for doing specific tests in problematic cases. For the effective execution of these investigations the posting of trained laboratory assistant or technician is important. These measures will also be of assistance in the antenatal clinics, epidemiological surveys and contact tracing. Besides, they help in the correct diagnosis, proper and adequate treatment and also in reducing the possibility of emergence of resistant strains of the organisms.

CONTACT TRACING

Complete eradication or uprooting of the ramifications of STD lies only in unfolding the source of reservoir of infection—an index case. This is one of the most vital functions of these clinics. This envisages seeking of detailed information from the patients about the possible sources or recipients of infection, and hopefully persuading them to attend the clinics for examination and treatment. General practitioners may also be persuaded to participate in this endeavor in addition to treating their own patients.

TREATMENT FACILITIES

Adequate supply of medicaments required for specific, effective and complete treatment of the STD patients and their contacts, helps to control and eventual eradication of the disease. Furthermore, the follow-up of the patients is a befitting complement to adequate and specific treatment, for it considerably assists in curtailing the morbidity and detecting treatment failures. The frequency and period of follow-up should, however, conform to the respective diseases.

EPIDEMIOLOGICAL SURVEYS

These clinics with the help of paramedical workers can conduct surveys to find out the prevalence of STD in the regions covered by them. This will help in the collection of statistics for the administrative planning and its execution.

HEALTH EDUCATION

It forms the backbone of control of STD. The involvement of the lay public is imperative. The awareness about the STD and sex in particular is very vital. A variety of methods can be used for the purpose, comprising public education, briefing at religious places, televisions, radios, documentaries and even a regular curriculum about sex at the school and college levels. The public and the patients should be encouraged to report and register at the regional health centers so that contact tracing can be facilitated.

Updating of physicians The practising physicians should be appraised of the quantum of STD and their effective up to date management through refresher courses conducted from time to time.

Updating of paramedical workers The paramedical workers should also be inducted to undergo similar training.

Orientation of the administrators and politicians. The need to change the attitude of those "at top" is very vital. In order to achieve this breakthrough, the organizing authority of health programs, should be made aware that a serious venereal disease problem exists or is likely to exist and that it should at least be assessed. This requires a change in attitude of the administrators, legislators and politicians. The change may come about from the influence of other members of the medical profession, from youth or other organizations within the country. It may result from prompting from outside government or nongovernment agencies like World Health Organization (WHO).

Funds The 'priority' control of STD should thus become a part accompaniment of health planning along with other communicable diseases. Hence, it envisages the allocation of adequate grants for its effective execution.

LEGISLATION

In many countries of the world, STDs are not included in the notifiable diseases. It is worthwhile making these diseases notifiable through a legislation. The existing legislation governing the prostitution needs modification so that it conforms to the rapidly changing socioeconomic pattern of the society of a respective country. This will considerably assist in the effective control of prostitution-a traditional reservoir of infection. Hence it will assist in worldwide control of STD.

VACCINES

Prophylactic vaccination of the susceptible group will be the best answer to control STDs. Efforts is being made at present to prepare a vaccine(s) against some of the STDs such as syphilis and gonorrhea.

Over and above, the international control of sexually transmitted diseases, now being mooted by the health administrators all over the world, should be reinforced with World Health Organization as the coordinating and the planning authority. HIV/acquire immunodeficiency syndrome (AIDS), is in particular, the focus for the future (*vide infra*).

Prevention of HIV/Acquired Immunodeficiency Syndrome (AIDS) Prevention

It is essential to keep following parameters in mind for the purpose:

1. ***Multiple sex partners:*** The risk of contracting HIV increases with the number of sexual partners. It is interesting to note that the first cases of AIDS, which was reported in homosexuals, admitted to having more than 100 sexual partners per year. A change in the lifestyle would obviously reduce the risk.
2. ***Pediatric AIDS:*** Generally occur early in life although some children have survived congenital infection for many years. Infected infants may serve as worldwide reservoirs of AIDS if they survive infancy, as in the case of hepatitis B.
3. ***HIV-infected mothers:*** They are not recommended to have children at present and pregnancy itself would appear to be a risk factor for seropositive mothers. A recent clinical trial demonstrated the efficacy of AZT in preventing transmission of HIV from the mother to the fetus. The incidence of HIV infection in the baby was reduced by 2/3rd. The regimen used in this trial included antenatal oral administration of AZT beginning at 14 to 34 weeks of gestation and continuing throughout pregnancy, followed by intrapartum IV AZT, and post-natal oral AZT to the infant for 6 weeks after delivery.
4. ***Blood and the bloods products:*** The spread of HIV through blood transfusion has virtually been eliminated, ever since the introduction of blood donor screening in many countries. It must be remembered that recently infected donors (latency) who have yet to develop antibodies will escape detection. There had also been recent reports of new virus isolates from patients serologically negative for HIV, yet who may have AIDS- related symptoms. Blood products such as factor VIII now undergo routine treatment, which appears to inactivate any HIV present effectively.

Development of Vaccines

An effective vaccine against HIV should elicit protection against both free virus and virus-infected cells. HIV neutralizing antibodies.

Several examples of retroviral infections like FeLV, suggest that neutralizing antibodies on its own may be protective. The observation that HIV-neutralizing antibodies do not prevent the progression of the disease and the induction of neutralizing antibodies in chimpanzees by HIV gp160 do not prevent infection by HIV argues against the possibility that neutralizing antibodies are sufficient for protection against infection by HIV. Individuals with high neutralizing antibody titers, however, seem to have a longer disease free interval. Cellular immune response may be important for protection and may take place through Tc cells, NK cells and ADCC mechanisms. The role of these mechanisms in the protection against HIV infection and their relevance for anti-HIV vaccination is not yet cleat.

Another obstacle to the development of an effective HIV vaccine may be the high genetic variability of HIV, which resides mainly in the env gene. In certain regions of the envelope gene, the variability may be as high as 50 percent. None the less, conserved regions exist in the gp120 and the gp41 region, which can be recognized by HIV sera and neutralizing antibodies can be induced with peptides representing these regions. The main types of approaches to an AIDS vaccine, should take cognizance of;

i. Live attenuated virus
ii. Inactivated virus
iii. Live recombinant viruses
iv. Synthetic peptides
v. Recombinant DNA products (gp120, gp160)
vi. Native envelope and/or core proteins
vii. Anti-idiotypes antibodies
viii. Passive immunization.

In view of the serious nature of the disease, and the ability of retroviruses to induce latency, it is unlikely that live attenuated/inactivated virus might ever be acceptable for human use. Live recombinant viruses such as vaccinia or adenovirus recombinant have been developed for HIV vaccination. They carry a high immunogenicity since virus replication result in large quantities of virus antigen. Both humoral and cellular immunity can be induced. A disadvantage of this approach is possible adverse effects observed after inoculation of vaccinia virus.

Synthetic peptides can be designed such that neutralizing and T cell epitopes can be included. The problems with synthetic peptides are related to the tertiary structures, which may be different from those of native proteins. Another promising approach is the production of recombinant viral antigens, especially the gene products of the env region, and the membrane associated p17 core protein. An alternative approach would be the use of anti-idiotype antibodies whose usefulness had been demonstrated against several infectious agents. Passive immunization may eventually be available for postexposure protection. To-date, it looks like that the best hope lies in an inactivated vaccine. Trials are being conducted with this vaccine in Thailand.

FURTHER READING

1. Baldwin HE. STD update: screening and therapeutic options. Int J Fertil Womens Med 2001;46:79-88.
2. Brown TJ, Yen-Moore A, Tyring SK. An overview of sexually transmitted diseases. Part I. J Am Acad Dermatol 1999;41:511-32.
3. Brown TJ, Yen-Moore A, Tyring SK. An overview of sexually transmitted diseases. Part II. J Am Acad Dermatol 1999;41:661-77.
4. Steele RW. Prevention and management of sexually transmitted diseases in adolescents. Adolesc Med 2000;11:315-26.
5. Thin RN. The legal framework covering the practice of genitourinary medicine in the UK: the venereal diseases Regulations. Int J STD AIDS 2001;12:701-4.

Appendices

Appendix 1: Gram's Staining

Prepare the smear from the material with the platinum loop, dry it and fix by passing over the flame.

Stain it with 0.5 percent methyl violet (crystal violet) solution for 20-30 seconds. Pour off the excess stain and add Lugol's iodine solution to wash away methyl violet. Allow the iodine to act for 30-60 seconds. Lugol's iodine is washed repeatedly with absolute alcohol until the color ceases to come out of the preparation. Later wash with water and counterstain with 0.5% safranin or neutral red for 30-60 seconds. Again wash with water and dry in between blotting papers.

Appendix 2: Wet Preparations

Wet preparations are useful to demonstrate *Candida albicans, Trichomonas vaginalis,* and *Treponema pallidum.* The method adopted for the collection of material, however, differs.

Candida albicans: For its demonstration, the scraping or discharge is collected on a clean glass slide, to which a drop of KOH (10-20 percent) is added. After a short interval, the slide is examined under the light microscope for the spores or pseudomycelia.

Trichomonas vaginalis: Here again the discharge is collected on a glass slide. It may either be instantly examined or a drop of normal saline is added before undertaking the examination. The morphology or motility can well be seen under light or dark-ground microscope.

Treponema pallidum: The material for the dark-ground examination is collected, by applying a cover slip to the lesions such as primary chancre, condylomata lata, mucous membrane patches after bathing them with normal saline. While the material from the lymph glands is collected-by injecting a little quantity of normal saline into the glands, and aspirating it. This material too is taken on a cover slip which is later placed on a thin slide and examined under the dark-ground microscope.

Appendix 3: Tissue Smear for Donovan Bodies

Preparation of smears: The ulcer is cleaned with saline soaked gauze. Its base is infiltrated with 1 percent lignocaine. Using a Bard-Parker knife, a piece of tissue is taken from the edge of the ulcer or from granulation tissue. Blood on the tissue is wiped off by gently soaking it on a blotting paper. The tissue is then squeezed with forceps and exudate is taken on a glass slide. This is dried in the air and fixed with methanol.

Staining of smears: It is then stained with 1 in 10 diluted Giemsa stain with a pH of 6.8. The Giemsa stain consists of stock Giemsa solution comprising 1 g of Giemsa powder and 66 ml each of methyl alcohol and glycerine. The diluted stain is kept on the slide for 10 minutes. The slide is washed with tap water, dried, and mounted with DPX mountant. Under the oil-immersion lens of the microscope the nuclei of the cells are deep blue, while the cytoplasm is pink. The Donovan bodies are identified as ovoid or bean-shaped 1.0-1.5 μ long and 0.5-0.7 μ thick. A pink material surrounds a blue bacillary body with dark blue or black chromatin inclusions. These organisms are seen inside cystic spaces or vacuoles in the large mononuclear cells'cytoplasm. The immature uncapsulated forms are either coccoid, diplococcoid, straight or curved rods with or without a closed safety-pin appearance, taking homogeneous or metachromatic stain.

Appendix 4: Dark-Ground Microscopy for *Treponema pallidum*

After the lesion is cleaned with saline, its surface is cleaned with gauze piece to obtain clear serum.

This is taken on three sides of a cover-slip and is pressed on a thin glass slide to spread it uniformly without any air bubbles. Excess serum is wiped with blotting paper. The edges of the cover slip are sealed with vaseline to prevent drying. A drop of oil is put over the cover slip, on the condenser of the microscope and under surface of the slide.

Treponema pallidum is identified as closely and regularly coiled, spiral, sluggishly motile, brilliantly bright organism. Movements of propulsion and change of shape namely angulation, buckling, undulation, looping, coil compression and expansion are considered diagnostic for syphilis.

Appendix 5: Genital Ulcers: Laboratory Investigations

- Gram stained smear for *Haemophilus ducreyi*
- Culture for *Haemophilus ducreyi*
- Dark-ground microscopy for *reponema pallidum*
- Serological tests for syphilis
- Tzanck smear for herpetic multinucleate giant cells
- Giemsa stained tissue smear for donovan bodies
- Histopathology and slow overnight Giemsa staining
- Screening for HIV infection.

Appendix 6: Chancroid: Newer Diagnostic Techniques

An endeavor to culture *Haemophilus ducreyi* forms an integral component of the battery of investigations undertaken for the diagnosis of genital sores. *H.ducreyi* is a fastidious microorganism, with varied nutritional requirements. Use of suboptimal media, improper collection and delayed inoculation further hinder recovery on culture. Although a variety of culture media, including fresh clotted human blood, and Müeller-Hinton media have been tried, none has provided an optimal growth. In the recent past, a combination of enriched gonococcal-agar base (GC-HgS) and enriched Müeller-Hinton (MH-HB) incorporated into a single biplate, has provided a high cultural yield of *H.ducreyi,* facilitating a definitive diagnosis of chancroid.

COMPOSITION

Gonococcal agar base + 1-2% hemoglobin + 5% fetal bovine serum + 10% coenzymes, vitamins, and amino acid (CVA) enrichment (GC - HgS) + vancomycin .

Müller-Hinton agar + 5% chocalatized horse blood + 10% CVA enrichment (MH-HB) + vancomycin.

Other Diagnostic Techniques

- Indirect immunofluorescence test using monoclonal antibodies directed against outer-membrane proteins of *H. ducreyi.*
- Radiolabelled DNA probes for *H. ducreyi.*
- Polymerase chain reaction to detect bacterial DNA in ulcer exudate/bubo aspirate.

Note: Vancomycin may be excluded if strains are suspected to be sensitive to this drug.

Appendix 7: Penicillinase Producing *Neisseria gonorrhoeae* (PPNG)

The emergence of strains of *Neisseria gonorrhoeae* resistant to penicillin and other antibiotics is now well-established. It, therefore, necessitates in depth understanding of 'its mechanism and emerging scenario of its current status. This requires setting up of surveillance centers to carry out gonococcal culture and antibiotic sensitivity testing, updating the recommendations for treatment, and follow-up, contact tracing, and enforcement of drug control measures to prevent irrational therapy.

Antibiotic resistance in *N. gonorrhoeae* may be controlled by genes on either chromosomes or plasmid. Chromosomal mediated resistance (CMR) results from mutations at several resistance loci. The CMR to penicillin is expressed through changes in the gonococcal cell-envelope. In general, CMR is partial and spreads slowly. Such resistance has been reported to various anti-microbial agents including penicillin, tetracyclines, cephalosporins, spectinomycin, thiamphenicol, rosoxacin, as well as newer fluoroquinolones.

The plasmid mediated resistance, was recorded initially in 1976, with the emergence of penicillinase producing *Neisseriae gonorrhoeae* (PPNG). The strains possess a resistance plasmid that codes for the enzyme beta-lactamase (penicillinase). This acts on the beta-lactam ring of penicillin molecule and converts it into inactive penicillinoic acid, thus destroying its antibiotic action. Some of the plasmids coding for antibiotic resistance require conjugative plasmids to enable them to move between the strains. The resistance is absolute, and spreads rapidly unlike CMR.

The diagnosis of penicillinase producing *N gonorrhoeae* requires meticulous culture sensitivity studies. All strains of *N. gonorrhoeae* showing inhibition less than 20 mm, with 10 IU penicillin disk should be investigated for penicillinase production. Several tests, namely below are helpful.

- Chromogenic cephalosporin test
- Acidometric test
- Rapid iodometric test

Should an endeavor to obviate such a situation be made, it is imperative to strictly adhere to the recommendations of Centre for Disease Control, Atlanta.

Appendix 8: Slow (Overnight) Giemsa Staining for Histopathological Sections

FIXATION OF THE TISSUE

The tissue is fixed in Zenker fluid or 10% formalin.

Embedding

The tissue is embedded in paraffin at 62°C. The temperature of the block is brought down by cooling. Sections are cut at 4 or 5 microns.

The solutions to be used are formulated as follows:

Giemsa stock solution		
Giemsa powder	1	g
Methyl alcohol	66	ml
Glycerine	66	ml
Working solution—Giemsa stain		
Stock Giemsa	0.5	ml
Methyl alcohol	1.5	ml
Distilled water	50	ml
Rosin stock solution		
White rosin	10	g
Absolute alcohol	100	ml
Working solution rosin		
Rosin stock solution		
95% alcohol	40	ml

Technique of Staining

Pass the tissue through:

1. Xylene and absolute alcohol for deparaffinization
2. Absolute alcohol
3. 95% alcohol
4. Iodine, and 5% sodium thiosulfate, if the tissue is zenker fixed
5. Wash well in running water
6. Rinse in distilled water

7. Place in working solution of Giemsa, 1% Stain overnight (4 PM to 9 AM next day)
8. Differetiate in 1% acetic acid until section resumes a purplish pink color. Check under the microscope
9. Give 2 changes in absolute alcohol
10. Give 2 changes in xylene
11. Mount in "Clarite" or "Permount" mountants.
12. Result:

Nucleus	:	blue
Cytoplasm and collagen	:	pink
Donovan bodies	:	purplish blue to pink

---

1. Sehgal VN, Jain MK. Tissue section Donovan bodies—identification through slow-Giemsa (overnight) technique. Dermatologica 1987; 174: 228-31.
2. Stary A. A correct samples for diagnostic tests in sexually transmitted diseases: which sample for which test? FEMS Immunol Med Microbiol 1999; 24: 455-9.

Appendix 9: Vocabulary of Generic and Trade Names of the Medicaments

Generic	*Trade namesh*
Ampicillin	Ampicillin, Ampilin, Ampilac, Synthocilin, Campicilin
Amoxycillin	Amoxycillin, Damoxy, Dinmox, Hipen, LMX-250/500
Benzathine penicillin	Benzyl penicillin, Longacillin, Pencom, Penidure, Pentids
Benzyl benzoate	Dermin lotion, Scabindon, Ascabiol
Chloramphenicol	Biophenicol, Chloromycetin, Enteromycetin, Phenimycin succinate, Vitamycetin
Cotrimaxazole	Septran, Bactrim, Cotrimaxazole
Demeclocycline hydrochloride	Ledermycin
Doxycycline	Biodoxi, Doxy-1, Microdox, Doxt, Ceedox-DT
Erythromycin	Erythrocin,Althrocin,Etomin,Eromed-333
Gamma benzene hexachloride	Ascabiol, Emscab, Scabex, Gamascab
Gentamicin	Gentamicin, Gentamicin, G-Mycin
Gentian violet	Gentian violet
Kanamycin	Kanamac, Kancin
Metronidazole	Flagyl, Largyl, Metrogyl, Metron
Nystatin cream	Mycostatin
Nystatin vaginal tablets	Mycostatin
Oxytetracycline	Oxytetracycline, Terramycin-SF
Podophyllum resin	Podowart Paint, Podowart-s Paint
Probenecid	Bencid
Procaine penicillin	Benzyl pencilin, Bistrepen, Bistrepen forte, Bistrepen paed.
Fortified with	Fortified procaine penicillin
Crystalline penicillin	Longacillin, Pencom
Spectinomycin	Trobicin
Spiramycin	Rovamycin forte
Streptomycin	Ambistryn-S
Sulphamethizole	Sulphamethizole
Tetracycline hydrochloride	Hostacyclin, Tetracycline, Achromycin, Tetracyl
Tetraethylthiuram	Tetmosol
Trichloracetic acid	Trichloracetic acid
Trimethoprim-sulphamethoxazole	Septran, Bectrim
Triple sulfonamide	Triple sulfa
Tinidazole	Tiniba, Tizole, Zil, Zoacide, Mobitide

HIV AND AIDS

Lamivudine + Stavudine + Nevirapine	Triomune-30/40
Lamivudine + Zidovudine + Nevirapine	Duovir-N
Lamivudine + Stavudine	Lamivir-S
Lamivudine + Zidovudine	Combivir, Duovir, Lamuzid
Nevirapine	Nevimune
Efavirenz	Efavir
Indinavir	Indivan
Stavudine	Stavir
Didanosine	Dinex
Lamivudine	Lamivir
Zidovudine	Retrovir, Zidovir, Zydowin, Ziv-100
Nevirapine	Navimune

1. IDR, Indian Drug Review. Mediworld publication, New Delhi. 2002; 8: (1).

Appendix 10: Center for Disease Control and Prevention (CDC) Guidelines for the Treatment of Sexually Transmitted Infection

UNCOMPLICATED GONOCOCCAL INFECTIONS OF THE CERVIX, URETHRA, AND RECTUM

Recommended Regimens*

Ceftriaxone 125 mg IM in a single dose

Or

Cefixime 400 mg orally in a single dose or 400 mg by suspension (200 mg/5 ml)

PLUS

Treatment for Chlamydia if Chlamydial infection is not ruled out

Alternative Regimens

Spectinomycin† 2 g in a single intramuscular (IM) dose

Or

Single-dose cephalosporin regimens

Other single dose cephalosporin regimens

ceftizoxime 500 mg IM; or

cefoxitin 2 g IM, administered with probenecid 1 g orally;

or cefotaxime 500 mg IM. Some evidence indicates that cefpodoxime 400 mg and cefuroxime axetil 1 g might be oral alternatives.

---

*These regimens are recommended for all adult and adolescent patients, regardless of travel history or sexual behavior.

†Spectinomycin is currently not available in the United States.

UNCOMPLICATED GONOCOCCAL INFECTIONS OF THE PHARYNX

Recommended Regimens*

Ceftriaxone 125 mg IM in a single dose

PLUS

Treatment of chlamydial infections if it is not ruled out.

Disseminated Gonococcal Infection (DGI)

Recommended Regimen

Ceftriaxone 1 g IM or IV every 24 hours

Alternative Regimens

Cefotaxime 1 g IV every 8 hours

Or

Ceftizoxime 1 g IV every 8 hours

Or

Spectinomycin† 2 g IM every 12 hour

Cefixime 400 mg orally twice daily

Or

Cefixime 400 mg by suspension (200 mg/5 ml) twice daily

Or

Cefpodoxime 400 mg orally twice daily.

Fluoroquinolones may be an alternative treatment option if antimicrobial susceptibility can be documented by culture. With use of nonculture tests to diagnose *N. gonorrhoeae* increasing and with local data on antimicrobial susceptibility less available, laboratories should maintain the capacity to conduct such testing or form partnerships with laboratories that can.

PELVIC INFLAMMATORY DISEASE (PID)

Parenteral Treatment

Parenteral and oral therapy appear to have similar clinical efficacy treating women with PID of mild or moderate severity. Clinical experience should guide decisions regarding transition to oral therapy, which usually can be initiated within 24 hours of clinical improvement.

---

*This regimen is recommended for all adult and adolescent patients, regardless of travel history or sexual behavior.

† A cephalosporin-based intravenous regimen is recommended for the initial treatment of DGI. This is particularly important when gonorrhea is detected at mucosal sites by nonculture tests. Spectinomycin is not currently available in the USA. Treatment should be continued for 24–48 hours after clinical improvement, at which time therapy may be switched to one of the following regimens to complete at least 1 week of antimicrobial therapy.

Recommended Parenteral Regimen A

Cefotetan 2 g IV every 12 hours

Or

Cefoxitin 2 g IV every 6 hours

Plus

Doxycycline 100 mg orally or IV every 12 hours

Recommmended Parenteral Regimen B

Clindamycin 900 mg IV every 8 hours

Plus

Gentamicin loading dose IV or IM (2 mg/kg of body weight), followed by a maintenance dose (1.5 mg/kg) every 8 hours. Single daily dosing may be substituted.

Alternative Parenteral Regimens

Ampicillin/Sulbactam 3 g IV every 6 hours

Plus

Doxycycline 100 mg orally or IV every 12 hours

Oral Treatment

Oral therapy can be considered for women with mild-to-moderately severe acute PID, as the clinical outcomes among women treated with oral therapy are similar to those treated with parenteral therapy. Women who do not respond to oral therapy within 72 hours should be reevaluated to confirm the diagnosis and should be administered parenteral therapy on either an outpatient or in-patient basis.

Recommended Oral Regimen

Ceftriaxone 250 mg IM in a single dose

Plus

Doxycycline 100 mg orally twice a day for 14 days

With or without

Metronidazole 500 mg orally twice a day for 14 days

Or

Cefoxitin 2 g IM in a single dose and **Probenecid**, 1 g orally administered concurrently in a single dose

Plus

Doxycycline 100 mg orally twice a day for 14 days

With or without

Metronidazole 500 mg orally twice a day for 14 days

Or

Other parenteral third-generation **cephalosporin** (e.g., **ceftizoxime** or **cefotaxime**)

Plus

Doxycycline 100 mg orally twice a day for 14 days

With or without

Metronidazole 500 mg orally twice a day for 14 days

Alternative Oral Regimens

If parenteral cephalosporin therapy is not feasible, use of fluoroquinolones (levofloxacin 500 mg orally once daily or ofloxacin 400 mg twice daily for 14 days) with or without metronidazole (500 mg orally twice daily for 14 days) may be considered if the community prevalence and individual risk (see "Gonococcal Infections in Adolescents and Adults" in Sexually Transmitted Disease Treatment Guidelines, 2006) of gonorrhea is low. Tests for gonorrhea must be performed prior to instituting therapy and the patient managed as follows if the test is positive:

- If NAAT test is positive, parenteral cephalosporin is recommended.
- If culture for gonorrhea is positive, treatment should be based on results of antimicrobial susceptibility. If isolate is QRNG, or antimicrobial susceptibility can not be assessed, parenteral cephalosporin is recommended.

Although information regarding other outpatient regimens is limited, amoxicillin/clavulanic acid and doxycycline or azithromycin with metronidazole has demonstrated short-term clinical cure. No data has been published regarding the use of oral cephalosporins for the treatment of PID.

CHANCROID

Recommended Regimens

1. Azithromycin 1 gm orally in a single dose
2. Ceftriaxone 250 mg, I/M in a single dose

Or

3. Ciprofloxacin 500 mg orally, twice a day for 3 days

Or

4. Erythromycin 500 mg base, three times a day for 7 days

Ciprofloxacin is contraindicated in pregnant and lactating women

Azithromycin and ceftriaxone have the advantage of single dose therapy

World wide several isolates with intermediate resistance to ciprofloxacin and erythromycin have been reported.

Safety and efficacy of azithromycin in pregnancy is not confirmed and ciprofloxacin is contraindicated during pregnancy and lactation.

EPIDIDYMITIS

Since empiric therapy is often initiated before laboratory tests are available, it is recommended that all patients receive ceftriaxone plus doxycycline for the initial therapy of epididymitis. Additional therapy may include a quinolone if acute epididymitis is not caused by gonorrhea (i.e., results from culture or nucleic acid amplification testing are negative for *N. gonorrhoeae*) or if the infection is most likely caused by enteric organisms.

Recommended Regimens

Ceftriaxone 250 mg IM in a single dose

PLUS

Doxycycline 100 mg orally twice a day for 10 days

For acute epididymitis most likely caused by enteric organisms or with negative gonococcal culture or nucleic acid amplification test

Ofloxacin 300 mg orally twice a day for 10 days

Or

Levofloxacin 500 mg orally once daily for 10 days

Severe Adverse Reactions to Penicillins or Cephalosporins

Immediate (30-60 minutes after administration) and accelerated (1-12 hours after administration) immunoglobin E mediated anaphylactic or urticarial reactions to cephalosporins are rare relative to those associated with penicillin. Reactions to first generation cephalosporins occur in approximately 5-10% of persons with a history of penicillin allergy, and occur less frequently in those administered third generation regimens. However, medical history and penicillin skin test results do not reliably predict the probability of allergic reactions to cephalosporins in those with history of penicillin allergy. Persons who can not tolerate cephalosporins should be treated with spectinomycin, if available. Because spectinomycin is not adequately effective against pharyngeal infections, patients who have suspected or known pharyngeal infection should have a pharyngeal culture evaluated 3-5 days after treatment to verify eradication of infection.

Since there are limited data regarding alternative regimens for treating gonorrhea among persons who have documented severe cephalosporin allergy, expert infectious diseases consultation is recommended; the best available treatment option is cephalosporin treatment following desensitization. If desensitization is not an option, azithromycin may be considered. Azithromycin 2 grams orally are effective against uncomplicated gonococcal infection, but concerns over emerging antimicrobial resistance to macrolides should restrict its use to limited circumstances.

FIRST CLINICAL EPISODE OF GENITAL HERPES +

Recommended Regimens*

Acyclovir 400 mg orally three times a day for 7–10 days

Or

Acyclovir 200 mg orally five times a day for 7–10 days

* Treatment might be extended if healing is incomplete after 10 days of therapy.

Or

Famciclovir 250 mg orally three times a day for 7–10 days

Or

Valacyclovir 1 g orally twice a day for 7–10 days

Established HSV-2 Infection

Recommended Regimens

Chronic suppressive therapy for recurrent genital herpes (>6 episodes/year)

Acyclovir 400 mg orally twice a day

Or

Famciclovir 250 mg orally twice a day

Or

Valacyclovir 500 mg orally once a day

Or

Valacyclovir 1.0 g orally once a day

Episodic Therapy for Recurrent Genital Herpes

Effective episodic treatment of recurrent herpes requires initiation of therapy within 1 day of lesion onset or during the prodrome that precedes some outbreaks. The patient should be provided with a supply of drug or a prescription for the medication with instructions to initiate treatment immediately when symptoms begin.

Recommended Regimens

Acyclovir **400 mg orally three times a day for 5 days**

Or

Acyclovir **800 mg orally twice a day for 5 days**

Or

Acyclovir **800 mg orally three times a day for 2 days**

Or

Famciclovir **125 mg orally twice daily for 5 days**

Or

Famciclovir **1000 mg orally twice daily for 1 day**

Or

Valacyclovir **500 mg orally twice a day for 3 days**

Or

Valacyclovir **1.0 g orally once a day for 5 days**

Severe Disease

Intravenous (IV) acyclovir therapy should be provided for patients who have severe HSV disease or complications that necessitate hospitalization (e.g., disseminated infection, pneumonitis, or hepatitis) or CNS complications (e.g., meningitis or encephalitis). The recommended regimen is acyclovir 5-10 mg/kg body weight IV every 8 hours for 2-7 days or until clinical improvement is observed, followed by oral antiviral therapy to complete at least 10 days of total therapy.

Recommended Regimens for Daily Suppressive Therapy in Persons Infected with HIV

Acyclovir 400-800 mg orally twice to three times a day

Or

Famciclovir 500 mg orally twice a day

Or

Valacyclovir 500 mg orally twice a day

Recommended Regimens for Episodic Infection in Persons Infected with HIV

Acyclovir 400 mg orally three times a day for 5-10 days

Or

Famciclovir 500 mg orally twice a day for 5-10 days

Or

Valacyclovir 1.0 grams orally twice a day for 5-10 days

Acyclovir, valacyclovir, and famciclovir are safe for use in immunocompromised patients in the doses recommended for treatment of genital herpes. For severe HSV disease, initiating therapy with acyclovir 5-10 mg/kg body weight IV every 8 hours might be necessary.

If lesions persist or recur in a patient receiving antiviral treatment, HSV resistance should be suspected and a viral isolate should be obtained for sensitivity testing. Such patients should be managed in consultation with an HIV specialist, and alternate therapy should be administered. All acyclovir-resistant strains are resistant to valacyclovir, and the majority is resistant to famciclovir. Foscarnet, 40 mg/kg body weight IV every 8 hours until clinical resolution is attained, is frequently effective for treatment of acyclovir-resistant genital herpes. Topical cidofovir gel 1% applied to the lesions once daily for 5 consecutive days also might be effective. This preparation is not commercially available and must be compounded at a pharmacy.

GRANULOMA INGUINALE

Recommended regimen

Doxycycline 100 mg orally, twice a day for 3 weeks and until all lesions have completely healed.

Alternative Regimen

Azithromycin 1 gm, orally once a wee for at least 3 weeks or until all lesions have completely healed

Or

Ciprofloxacin 750 mg twice a day, orally at least for 3 weeks or until all lesions have completely healed

Or

Erythromycin 500 mg orally, 4 times a day, at least for 3 weeks or until all lesions have completely healed

Or

Trimethoprim-sulfamethoxazole, one double strength (160-800 mg) tablet orally twice a day for at least 3 weeks or until all lesions have healed completely.

Some specialists recommend addition of aminoglycoside (gentamicin 1mg/kg, every 8 hourly) to these regimens if improvement is not evident with these regimens within first few days of therapy.

LYMPHOGRANULOMA VENEREUM

Recommended regimen

Doxycycline 100 mg twice a day for 21 days

Or

Erythromycin 500 mg 4 times a day for 21 days

SYPHILIS

Primary and Secondary syphilis for adults

Benzathine Penicillin G 2.4 mega unit, by single intramuscular injection

Recommended regimen for children

Benzathine penicillin 50,000 units/kg IM up to the total adult dose of 2.4 million units in a single dose.

Latent Syphilis

Benzathine penicillin 2.4 million units IM in a single dose

Late latent syphilis or syphilis of unknown duration

Benzathine penicillin 7.2 million units, administered as 3 doses of 2.4 million units IM each at 1 week interval

Recommended regimen for children

Early Latent Syphilis

Benzathine penicillin 50, 000 units/kg IM, up to the adult dose of 2.4 million units in a single dose

Late Latent Syphilis or Syphilis of Unknown Duration

Benzathine Penicillin G 50,000 units/kg/IM up to the adult dose of 2.4 million units administered as 3 doses at 1 week interwal (total 150,000 units/kg upto the adult total dose of 7.2 million units.

Tertiary Syphilis

Benzathine Penicillin G 7.2 million units, total administered as 3 doses of 2.4 million units IM each at 1 week interval.

Neurosyphilis

Aqueous crystalline penicillin G 18-24 million units per day administered as 3-4 million units IV every 4 hours or continuous infusion for 10-14 days.

Alternative regimens

Procaine Penicillin 2.4 million units IM once daily

Plus

Probenecid 500 mg orally 4 times aday both for 10-14 days.

Index